CURL TALK

CURL TALK

Everything You Need to Know

to Love and Care for Your Curly,

Kinky, Wavy, or Frizzy Hair

OUIDAD

with Jennifer Schonbrunn Hinkle

 THREE RIVERS PRESS · NEW YORK

Published by Three Rivers Press, New York, New York.
Member of the Crown Publishing Group,
a division of Random House, Inc.

www.randomhouse.com

THREE RIVERS PRESS and the Tugboat design
are registered trademarks of Random House, Inc.

Printed in the United States of America

DESIGN BY KAREN MINSTER

*Special thanks to Mark Babushkin, photographer, and
Michael Evanston, illustrator, for their contributions to the book.*

Library of Congress Cataloging-in-Publication Data
Ouidad.
Curl talk: everything you need to know to love and care for your
curly, kinky, wavy, or frizzy hair / by Ouidad, with Jennifer
Schonbrunn Hinkle.—1st ed.
1. Hair—Care and hygiene.   I. Hinkle, Jennifer Schonbrunn.
II. Title.
RL91.0955 2002
646.7′24—dc21   2002018811

ISBN 0-609-80837-0

10   9   8   7   6   5   4

FIRST PAPERBACK EDITION

This book is dedicated to the memory of my parents,
Antoinette and John Stephen;
to Peter, P.J., and Sondriel, with all my love;
and to all the women over the years
who have given me the honor of caring for their curls
and learning from them.

Acknowledgments

Completing this book has been an educational process for me and a refresher course in all that I have learned and taught throughout the years. It has involved an orchestra of people: I am grateful to the chemists and stylists who have worked with me for many years on my techniques and products; to Christo, my salon creative director, who continually challenges me in our constant discussions about hair; to my sister, Susan, who provided me with a head of hair that I thought I'd never get out from under; and to the many dermatologists whom I've given a hard time about women and hair loss.

Then there is my team—the hairdressers that carefully read various chapters for me to make sure I had it all right. If there are errors in this book, they are all mine; if it is accurate, it is thanks to the generosity of these people. My thanks to: Christo, Anna Daniel, Vincent Voorhees, Ayanna Augustine, Robert Nieves Jr., Latesha Campbell, Anila Poreci, Mioara Grecu, and to all my clients that shared their personal hair stories with me.

Within the orchestra there are always the soloists: Thank you to my wonderful husband and business partner, Peter, who is always ready to hear and give 100 percent to our latest and greatest new idea; to Jennifer Hinkle, the beauty editor and writer who has worked on all my projects, website material, brochures, and this book with me—she knows just how to capture my voice and just when to say, "Wait—what does that mean?"—her patience and diligence are overwhelming, and she makes the best sweets to boot.

Finally, there is my family: Peter John Wise, still the love of my life after more than twenty years; P.J., our thirteen-year-old son, who is extremely bright and always keeps us guessing; and Sondriel, our eleven-year-old daughter, who keeps saying, "Can you curl my hair more?" and has developed some of her own talents with hair. Thank you all for putting up with me!

I am especially humbled by all the generations of women with curly hair who have found my expertise has been useful throughout the years. It is a true honor to help you understand a bit better what happens to this head called curls.

Contents

Foreword

Did you know 60 percent of American women have some form of curly hair? It's a little-known fact concealed by straightening, relaxing, softening, perming, ironing, blow-drying, and gallons of styling products. The truth is, natural curls are a gift! What other tresses boast such enviable body, movement, and versatility?

Forget spending hours wrestling with your curls! Adopt my philosophy—choose the path of least resistance. That means work *with* your hair type, don't fight it. I've yet to meet a winner in that battle. At the end of the day, it's still a personal decision. My goal is to help people love their locks and find a style that suits their look and lifestyle without damaging their hair—that's all that matters.

So let those poor souls with straight hair get carpal tunnel syndrome from curling-iron abuse—we curly girls are ready to celebrate what we've got, and I am here to lead the way!

WHO AM I?

Once you get past my difficult-to-pronounce name (Ouidad—"wee-dod"), the first thing you should know is, I have extremely curly hair, so this topic is near and dear to my heart.

I didn't wake up one morning and feel a need to write this book. I have lived this topic since I was a child.

As a kid, my sister had championship curly hair. It was dense with such tight ringlets that you could have made three voluminous wigs out of it. And believe me, I seriously considered this when I was awakened each morning at five to the irritating whir of my sister's blow-dryer. For nearly ninety minutes, she would straighten her hair until she achieved a giant helmet head. My greatest ammunition against her? A spray bottle of water!

Once she had finished her hair ritual, we'd leave for school—she with her blown-out "wings," and me with curly, thick, and big long hair. We were teased mercilessly by our classmates who apparently preferred a stick-straight *Mod Squad* look. My response, as a consummate tomboy, was to beat up anyone who insulted us. I quickly realized this was not the best approach and began attacking the root of the problem: curly hair.

I started experimenting with different ways to tame curls. I had the perfect audience—my own family of wavy manes. My family comes from Lebanon, yet surprisingly we don't all have typically thick, wiry Middle Eastern tresses. My mom had coarse, dense curls, while my dad had less coarse curly waves and my brothers have fine, thick curls. (You already know my sister's situation.) Styling and working with our various hair types became fun. My family soon came to respect my opinions, and they'd listen to anything I had to say. Wow—such power!

When my family moved to Providence, Rhode Island, in 1973, I complemented my studies with a job at a local salon. In the summertime, I sought out apprenticeships all over

Europe. I began at Antonio's in Rome, where I mastered the art of clipping and working with shears, particularly on coarse and curly hair. The following summer I worked in Paris under renowned hairdresser Alexander Zauri, where we styled hair and makeup for high-profile clients, including Christian Dior and Yves Saint Laurent. My third summer took me to London through a hairdresser-training program—but I never returned to the States. I remained in England and established my career there, working with celebrity stylist Danny Valesco. After doing the hair for the original production of *Evita* in London, I decided to join Valesco's team and help launch the show in New York in 1978.

It was an exhilarating time for the beauty industry as well as for me personally. I continued to develop my career working with this same group of stylists, doing hair and makeup for Broadway shows, advertising agencies, and fashion magazines. I would always work on the curly heads—they were the most natural to me. Over the next five years, I styled hair for many major ad campaigns and fashion shoots, including Ralph Lauren, Calvin Klein, The Gap, Revlon, American Express, and Benetton. My expertise with curly hair was recognized beyond the advertising world in 1979, 1980, and 1981 when I won the North American Hairstyling Awards for Best Stylist in the United States.

In 1982 I met my husband, Peter. Despite his naturally straight hair, we decided to get married. Our next decision was to start a business—it would be either in the restaurant world, in which he was well established, or in my realm, the beauty industry. Both of us were strong minded and driven, so we did the only thing we could do—flip a coin. Heads (of course) a salon, tails a restaurant. As luck would have it, the

Ouidad Salon was born. At age twenty-six, we embarked on this exciting venture—and our lives haven't stopped changing since.

Within a few years, the Ouidad Salon became the mecca of curly hair. Clients were visiting me in New York from all over the world. Stylists in Italy, England, Saudi Arabia, Israel, Brazil, Argentina, Egypt, and beyond heard about my special curly-hair-cutting technique and referred their clients to me. The "curly grapevine" was born! When I'd hear about this international source of customers, I'd think to myself, "This is great! I've done something great." I was helping people from across the globe to look and feel good about their hair. People constantly tell me I've changed their lives. No matter how often I hear that, I can't help but smile—a continual reminder of what my purpose is in life: to make every curly-headed person understand and love their fabulous hair.

Thanks to this worldwide network of clients, the Ouidad Salon has been thriving since its inception. But as any good hairdresser knows, a great cut is only half the equation for beautiful curls. The right products are essential not only to initially creating a look but to at-home styling. I hadn't found what I considered the perfect curly hair products, so I spent many years mixing and layering various brands to tame my clients' and my own curly hair. Finally, I began experimenting by making my own products from scratch. After successfully testing the formulas on friends and family, I decided to share my research and development with clients. By 1982 I was preparing my own curly hair elixir, Deep Treatment, for our salon customers on an individual basis and quickly found the demand was outpacing the supply. Within six years, I publicly introduced Deep Treatment to customers and the press,

receiving rave reviews, including a feature story in *Town &
Country* magazine and appearances on *Sally Jessy Raphael,*
CNN, *Eyewitness News, Later Today,* and Univision Español.
This success encouraged me to return to the laboratory, where
I created Clear Shampoo, Balancing Rinse, and my collection
of signature products.

A successful business, a wonderful husband and business
partner, plus two terrific kids—sounds like I have it all! On
paper it looks easy, but day-to-day life is a tremendous jug-
gling routine. First of all, I live in Connecticut, over an hour
away from my Manhattan salon. Instead of facing the lengthy
commute each day, I spend three to four days (and nights) a
week in New York City, and the balance at the company's cor-
porate offices near our home. It's exhausting and sometimes
lonely, but somehow it works. While I am in Manhattan
whizzing among salon clients, photo shoots, and magazine
interviews, my husband oversees the care of our kids, Peter
(with straight hair like his dad) and Sondriel (with slightly
wavy hair—I have to *pin-curl* it for real curls!) when he's not
running our product division, the mail-order business, and
the website. We define the term *partnership!*

Just a few years ago I headed back to the lab and created
Ouidad Climate Control, a humidity-fighting styling lotion,
which was awarded Best De-Frizzer by *Allure* magazine in
1999. This product, along with the entire collection of Ouidad
products, was designed and produced without the use of animal testing—a practice we fiercely uphold in all levels of
development. Since then we've developed and launched
Ouidad Curl Quencher Shampoo, designed for extremely
dehydrated and chemically thirsty curls, and the companion
moisturizing Curl Quencher Conditioner.

In between cutting hair, creating new products, conducting press interviews, and working with Peter on the business itself, it struck me that there are still many people out there who are at loose ends with their curls. I am proud of my product line and cutting techniques that allow people to manage and truly adore their curls, but we have so many more people to reach. There is a wide gap between this group and the people who still spend hours with a blow-dryer, flat iron, and way too much silicone gel, coaxing their wavy locks straight. This book is for those of you who need to understand how curls work, how *your* curls work, and how to make peace with those seemingly untamable tresses.

For the past twenty-five years, I've had the privilege of working in the beauty industry with women and men of all walks of life, including celebrities, heads of state, fashion designers, professional women, friends, and of course my family. No matter how famous, beautiful, or wealthy these people are, a healthy head of curls links them together. Top women's magazines such as *Elle, Harper's Bazaar, Allure,* and *Vogue* now refer to me as "a curl's best friend," and that's how I want you to use this book. It's a guide and a friend— your curls are not the enemy, and this is not a war. I'm determined to help you love your curls!

CURL TALK

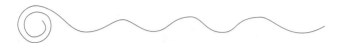

Anecdote: *This letter is one of many stories I hear over and over from my clients . . .*

Dear Ouidad,

I came from the Middle East to the United States in my midteens. I had big eyes and a big nose, full lips, and a huge, thick head of curls. I couldn't speak the language properly, and my high school and college peers were constantly making fun of my big hair. It was a difficult time, being a foreigner and having no friends. I took to ironing my hair on a daily basis to be accepted—I didn't even attend classes when it rained. I was studying medicine, but my hair problems were far more challenging than my schoolwork. I've been practicing medicine for over seven years but only discovered you recently. Now I'm free of my hair insecurities! Where were you when I was in college?

Gratefully,

Jane W., North Carolina

Introduction

The Curly Legacy

VIVE LE CURL

While women of the French Revolution, the Industrial Revolution, and the Sexual Revolution were working toward an enlightened society, they were beating their curls into submission. Instead of allowing tresses to remain in their naturally wavy state, a wide range of salves, irons, and rollers were employed to reshape every strand, either flattening natural curls or creating artificial ones.

Marie Antoinette is a great example. She and her eighteenth-century gal pals favored painstakingly perfect ringlets, yet dismissed their own source of curls, donning elaborate wigs instead. American southern belles of the Civil War era spent hours primping to create a similar look with their own hair—remember Scarlett O'Hara? With time, longer locks were replaced by more practical lengths that also exposed more natural curls. At the beginning of the twentieth century, close-cropped, wavy styles gained popularity as the flappers came into vogue.

As Hollywood blossomed, so did a look of starlet chic. The silver screen of the 1930s and 1940s glamorized Veronica Lake's demure finger waves and Rita Hayworth's seductive swirls, celebrating the curl yet perpetuating our need to manipulate and conceal their natural look. The message was that curls were socially acceptable as long as they were polished and controlled.

The late twentieth century saw a love-hate relationship with the curl. Natural waves were often ironed out on an actual ironing board (imagine Barbra Streisand in *The Way We Were*), only to be set on rollers for volume or to flip the ends, mimicking the stylish bobs of Grace Kelly and Jacqueline Kennedy Onassis. Others took cues from fashion designers who had fallen in love with the Afro. These voluminous, unabashed curls marked a breakthrough, both on the runway and on the street. A third style mimicked the tousled tendrils of sex symbol Brigitte Bardot, striking a balance between the highly overcoifed and the shockingly natural.

The 1970s also experienced a 'do dichotomy—the artificial feathered coif of Farrah Fawcett-Majors alongside the kinky curls of people like actress Jacqueline Bisset and singer Stevie Nicks. While *Charlie's Angels* wannabes were tied to their blow-dryers and paddle brushes, fans of Jane Fonda in *Klute* fluffed their locks with a pick comb. Permanent waves were becoming a popular request at salons, and those of us with real curls began to breathe a sigh of relief.

By the 1980s, curly hair was not only "in" but the focus of an important styling-aid invention: mousse. Many of us recall this revolutionary foam that encouraged our curls to remain springy and full (not to mention that awful "crunchy" stiffness). Alas, mousse was not the ideal curly hair helper, but it was one of the first products designed to enhance, not suppress, curls.

The 1980s and 1990s marked a distinct change in how we thought about hair. Instead of choosing a hairstyle and forcing locks into a specific shape, stylists encouraged women to follow the natural texture of their hair. Women were investing in hair*cuts* and styling products to enhance what they had, instead of heated appliances to redirect strands into unnatural shapes.

Now that we've entered the twenty-first century, beauty gurus do not prescribe a set hairstyle for each season. While each year may present innovative cutting techniques and styling aids, the bottom line is the individual. Women with curly hair are showing it off, thanks to terrific role models such as Debra Messing, Sarah Jessica Parker, Nicole Kidman, Julia Louis-Dreyfus, Julianna Margulies, Kate Hudson, Keri Russell, and Melina Kanakaredes.

Understanding Your Hair

CURLY HAIR CATEGORIES
(The Nine Lives of Curly Hair)

All curls are *not* created equal, which means there is no universal regimen that works for every type of wave. Therefore, it's essential to identify your hair's texture correctly in order to treat it right. After all, you wouldn't wash your face with dishwashing liquid or polish your nails with housepaint. Knowledge is power, so get to know your curls. Once you're familiar with your hair's personality, you'll know how to anticipate its mood swings and be able to control and prevent outbursts. A curl's best friend is awareness.

The following section outlines the various curl widths, textures, and conditions. Most manes contain a combination of each category—for example, one person may have fine, loose waves in the back with medium, coarser curls in the front— and each section needs slightly different care. Most of the time, we are so focused on its overall appearance that we don't take time to examine our hair in sections. If you study your own hair carefully, you'll be able to spot the various curl patterns and understand its unique language. As I always tell my clients, "Listen to your hair. It speaks to you." It may seem like a lot of work, but the payoff is huge. A healthy, well-tended head of curls is what turns straight-haired people green with envy. Need I say more?

So scan the following section for the characteristics that best describe your hair. As you read the book, mix and match the advice about styling products, cleansing, conditioning, and cuts to determine the best routine for your unique set of curls.

CURL PATTERNS

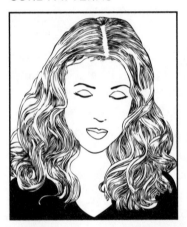

∗LOOSE: This soft, less defined curl features big, shiny waves approximately two inches wide. Sarah Jessica Parker, Julia Roberts, Heather Graham, and Ananda Lewis are the poster children for this category. When loose waves are cut short, they tend to look straighter, and they become curlier with length. But longer styles may weigh down a small face or diminish natural body, so keep this in mind when choosing a cut. While this curl pattern is easiest to straighten, don't be tempted to do it daily— even gentle waves are vulnerable to dehydration and heat damage.

∗CURLY: Your "classic" curls fall into tendrils one to one and a half inches wide. Your mane boasts lots of volume that may fool you into thinking your hair is coarse. Don't slip into this trap! Chances are, your tresses are fine and delicate and require tender care. The spiraled position forces the cuticle (the outer, protective layer of hair) to stay open and vulnerable to dehydrating forces that penetrate and rob the hair of its necessary moisture. This type of curl is tighter when cut short, and it transforms into looser spirals when worn longer. Many people who fall

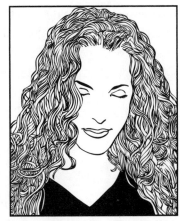

into this category bemoan the fact that they always look "too cute" or childish. Actresses such as Debra Messing, Julia Louis-Dreyfus, Julianna Margulies, Keri Russell, and Melina Kanakaredes remind us that this type of curl can in fact look sexy and sophisticated.

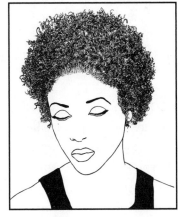

*KINKY: These tiny ringlets of an inch or less in diameter are probably the most fragile of all three categories. Like medium curls, the tightly coiled shape leaves the cuticle susceptible to dryness and damage from heat styling, chemical processes, the sun, pollution, and artificial air.

Tight curls fall into several patterns. When stretched out, you may see an S shape, a loose, reverse S like a Z, or both. The looser the curl pattern, the more moisture the hair has retained—although it's never enough. Hair in this category is often chemically straightened or softened, which demands extra care and maintenance. Angela Bassett, Halle Berry, Diana Ross, Carmen Ejogo, and Macy Gray's signature curls prove that proper styling, frequent deep conditioning treatments, and the right cut will keep that Bride of Frankenstein look at bay.

TEXTURES

*FINE: The biggest surprise my clients find out about their hair is that almost 99 percent of them have baby-fine locks. Contrary to popular belief, curly hair is often fine and quite delicate—no matter how voluminous or tightly spiraled. People frequently mistake density for coarseness, which leads to improper and harsh treatment. Care for your silky curls with a light touch—steer clear of thick styling gels and creams, silicones, and moisturizing formulas that contain oils. By applying lightweight products to your hair, you'll allow your fine curls to reveal their natural shape and spring.

*COARSE: These strands are thicker in diameter than fine hair and are much more resilient to damage. Curly hair is usually fine—coarse hair is typically found on the straighter hair of Asians and Native Americans. (Remember Pocahontas and her long smooth braids?) Sometimes mature women with gray hair will also find their tresses have become coarser. The cuticle of coarse hair stays closed, which keeps out frizz-causing moisture, flyaways, and split ends. While this hair texture may sound like a dream, it's actually so thick and heavy that curled sets rarely stay in.

CONDITION

*FRIZZY: Frizz is created when hair lacks its own internal weight. The spiraled pattern of each curly strand forces the cuticle to stay open, inviting dehydrating forces such as heated styling implements, the sun, and dry artificial air to rob the hair's inner segment of moisture and nutrients. The hair shaft is then virtually weightless, allowing tiny baby hairs to float away from the cuticle, creating that fuzzy halo effect. Well-conditioned and hydrated hair possesses inner weight that prevents flyaways, fostered by a closed cuticle, thus sealing the hair shaft off from a ruffled cuticle and the resulting frizz. The best way to eliminate frizz is to dry your hair naturally. Nature (read: water) is the best defense against dehydrated hair.

*DRY: By now, you've learned that curly hair is prone to dehydration. A perpetually open cuticle is a magnet for moisture-sappers such as harsh cleansers, heat styling, and environmental forces like wind and sun. A dry mane acts "tense"—strands don't relax and fall into healthy curl patterns. If you spend lots of time outside or are addicted to heat styling, weekly or biweekly deep conditioning treatments are vital to maintaining a beautiful set of curls.

*BRITTLE: Brittle tresses are most likely fragile from repeated permanent hair coloring, straightening chemicals, and excessive styling-product buildup. Just as you cleanse your face of makeup and dirt to prevent clogged pores, you must rid your hair of outside elements, such as silicones, waxes, and oils, that may stifle the hair shaft. Styling is a real challenge with brittle hair because it doesn't want to fall into a shape—it behaves lifelessly despite careful blow-drying or use of a curling iron. Give your hair a vacation from any chemical processes, and treat it to weekly conditioning treatments to restore its lost moisture and nutrients and rebuild its strength. Fortunately, this level of damage is rare.

∗SPLIT ENDS: Every mane—curly, straight, short, long—is susceptible to split ends. Strands become dry and "empty" from a variety of assaults, including the environment, frequent heat styling, and harsh cleansers. In this condition, the cuticle remains open and feathery. These tiny raised layers are actually split ends, also called flyaways. They are weightless and lift away from the cuticle, creating that halo of frizz. Contrary to popular belief, split ends are found all over the hair and *cannot* be fixed with cutting. The best treatment for split ends is to feed your hair, just like your skin. A nourished hair shaft will have enough internal weight to keep the cuticle closed so that each curl is smooth. Clearly, trimming split ends is not an option—you might as well shave your head. Since split ends can appear anywhere, frequent deep conditioning is the only way to prevent them. *Note:* You'll see the most flyaways in the winter, when the hair is prone to extreme dryness. For a quick fix, spray your tresses with a leave-in conditioner to quench their thirst.

What about humidity? Why does moisture wreak havoc on dry hair? The typical curly hair shaft is either empty or full of gaps where moisture and nutrients have escaped. Humidity fills the strands with moisture, forcing the cuticle to bulge open, creating a ruffled effect from the tiny baby hairs lifting along the hair shaft. The only kind of "good" moisture is the kind that remains self-contained within the hair shaft.

Why is it harder to hide frizz on curly hair? The corkscrew shape of each wave is predisposed to the frizzy effect (as described above), whereas on straight hair there's a single surface that can be flattened out with heavy styling products that would spoil the flow of natural curls.

MYTH: *The only way to prevent frizz is to use silicone-based products.*

TRUTH: Silicone is like hot fudge—it's best in small doses. Silicone creates a barrier between your hair and the elements, so in one way strands are protected from frizz-inducing rain, humidity, and perspiration. Unfortunately, silicone also smothers the hair's cuticle, preventing it from "breathing." If silicone products are used too often, the strands will become weak and limp and won't be able to form healthy, vibrant curls. Resort to silicone for emergencies, when you don't have time to style your hair properly.

MYTH: *Curly hair is always dry, so always choose moisturizing shampoos, conditioners, and stylers.*

TRUTH: While curly hair is prone to dryness, you should rehydrate your locks carefully. Many moisturizing products use oils and waxes to lend hair a smooth, silky texture. Your hair may feel less dry, but it will be difficult to style. These ingredients are too heavy and occlusive for curly tresses. By weighing down each strand and clogging the cuticle, your hair can't "breathe" and reveal its natural curl pattern. Look for products that contain cetrimonium chloride (vegetable), panthenol/pro-vitamin B5, and wheat amino acids to truly restore your hair's moisture. Don't be lured by Grandma's myth that olive oil is a great hair hydrator. Not only is it messy, but it will suffocate your hair shaft much like heavy styling aids.

MYTH: *Use a flat iron to get rid of frizz.*
TRUTH: Why not hold a match to your hair? Heat implements such as curling and flat irons singe the cuticle—and damage to this segment renders far more long-term damage and immediate frizz than blow-drying.

MYTH: *Split ends occur when the tips of your hair break apart.*
TRUTH: Surprise! Split ends are synonymous with flyaways and can occur in any section of the hair: the crown, the bangs, the sides, the nape, and—yes—the ends. As I mentioned earlier, split ends are the tiny baby hairs that lift away from the cuticle when the hair shaft is depleted and weightless. When your strands are dry, there aren't any nutrients to give them substance, so they float away from the cuticle, causing that dreaded ruffled, frizzy effect.

Don't be fooled . . . Hot oil treatments claiming to seal and repair split ends merely provide a temporary and incomplete service. Oils may smooth frizzy hair for a few hours, but they cannot permanently tame those flyaways. Oil will only perpetuate the problem by cutting the hair shaft off from valuable nutrients and moisture and causing the hair to become sticky with oily residue. Shrewd marketing causes consumers to believe split ends appear only on the tips of the hair, and that these forked hairs can be re-fused with their magical elixirs. Yes, it's too good to be true!

COMMON FRUSTRATIONS

Every day I hear variations on the same curly hair woes. Here are the top ten:

> "I spend an hour blow-drying and styling my hair, and then five minutes after I'm outside, it becomes frizzy. All my work was for nothing!"
>
> "I never feel finished."
>
> "I always look upset." (emotional tress stress)
>
> "I lost my boyfriend over my hair—he couldn't run his hands through my hair without getting caught in tangles."
>
> "Curly hair is so unpredictable."
>
> "It's uncontrollable!"
>
> "I look like Shirley Temple."
>
> "I look like I'm wearing a mop!"
>
> "I don't look professional."
>
> "I look 'wild,' and people view me as a 'wild' person."

The Care and Feeding of Curly Hair

"Ouidad, how do I handle my curly hair?"

As little as possible! Minimize contact with a wavy mane to maintain gorgeous, well-formed spirals. The key to beautiful curls is to position tresses while they're wet and then *leave them alone*. Once curls are dry, excessive primping (including finger-combing) will separate the curls, ruining the natural "puzzle piece" flow of your hair, resulting in frizz and uneven volume. Proper cleansing, regular conditioning, and deep nourishing treatments are the best insurance policy for smooth, vibrant curls. No matter how skilled you are at styling, dry and damaged hair will not produce beautiful, even waves.

If your hair is dull, damaged, dirty, or greasy, it won't matter how fabulous your haircut is—no one will notice it. People are distracted by unhealthy, frazzled hair. My clients and models and I are constantly asked how we keep our curls so healthy looking with our busy lives. It's simple: Feed! Feed! Feed! The beauty-magazine editors are always consulting me about healthy shiny curls, and I tell them: Feed! Feed! Feed!

This section provides a lot of information, techniques, and choices—but don't feel overwhelmed. Once you've practiced using my tips and tricks, they will become second nature. At that point, you'll realize that your daily regimen can be defined in three easy steps:

1. Cleanse and moisturize
2. Detangle and seal
3. Style, dry, and finish

I'm going to teach you and supply you with the ammunition you need to keep your hair healthy, soft, and gorgeous. Being well informed is your key to success!

SHAMPOO 101

Let's talk basics. Washing your hair rinses away dirt and oils and returns moisture to your hair. When you don't shampoo frequently enough, the secretion of oils combined with styling products and other debris from the environment will block your hair follicles and prevent vital nutrients from reaching the hair and scalp. This will cause dryness and a dulled appearance. Imagine this: After using olive oil in your salad, you placed the bottle on your kitchen counter, then sat down to eat. By the time you're cleaning up after dinner, the ring that the bottle left behind has already collected a fine layer of dust and impurities. Imagine the level of debris that would gather after a few days. Now imagine the countertop is your hair! Okay, I've made my point.

Don't forget, almost 70 percent of our bodies are made of water. Clogging the follicles with debris will slow down the process by which this element is replenished. I find that when clients don't shampoo often enough, not only are they suffocating their hair, but their follicles fill with oily white flakes and emit a very unpleasant odor. Ugh!

TO SHAMPOO OR NOT TO SHAMPOO: HOW OFTEN IS OFTEN ENOUGH?

We all need to shampoo our hair on a regular basis—but what is a regular basis for *your* hair? To set the record straight, it isn't necessary to shampoo daily, although this is a matter of personal preference. In the past, we would read through a beauty magazine and determine our cleansing schedule based on whether our hair type was normal, oily, or dry, but it's not that simple. Some scalps have all three conditions. So how do you handle that? Your hair texture and styling techniques will play a large role in setting a shampoo regimen, as I explain below.

*LOOSE: Because the structure of your hair is fairly coarse and strong, you can shampoo as often as four to five times a week, although I recommend less. As with all curls, use a low-pH shampoo.

*CURLY: Shampoo every second or third day with a gentle moisturizing shampoo. This category requires constant hydration—dryness will cause it to frizz and break. It's still important to rinse it daily with warm water, then follow with a detangling rinse on the ends to keep the hair moist and to revive your curls. I myself have medium curls, and I find that daily shampooing frizzes my hair. My hair looks best the day after I wash it. By the third day, I lose my curl pattern, and the life disappears from it. To freshen my curls and remove product buildup, I rinse my hair daily.

*KINKY: Shampoo these tight, fragile curls once a week; or twice, if you are especially active. I find this type of hair always looks and feels the driest when it needs a good shampoo. Remember, shampooing is a hydrating process because water is the most essential moisturizer. Make sure that you use a very mild, protein-based shampoo with natural ingredients. Don't forget, this type of hair is very fine and delicate—don't be fooled by its large visual appearance. Extra-gentle, nutrient-rich shampoos are a must—look for formulas with glycerin, sulfur, and carotene. If your hair is also very coarse, each strand has a larger-than-average diameter and a tendency to spring away from the scalp. I recommend my Curl Quencher Shampoo or one like it with extra humectants to moisturize and add weight, so curls are more defined and controlled.

SKIPPING A DAY

On days you do not shampoo, simply rinse the hair with warm water and apply a leave-in conditioner to detangle. Even the sweat from exercise can be rinsed with water alone. However, if the natural oils and sebum in your hair build up at a fast rate, you may choose to suds up daily.

SHAMPOO SHOPPING

Finding a good shampoo for your specific hair needs is no easy feat amid so many promising products. Twelve years ago I said the heck with it and took the extreme path. I studied chemistry to find out for myself what works best on various hair types, then created my own formulas. I was motivated by selfish reasons—developing my business into a curly hair empire! I'll give you the shortcut: Look for a gentle shampoo with a low pH of 6.6 to 6.8 designed for daily use (close to 7, the neutral pH level of bottled water), or consider formulas created for chemically processed or color-treated hair. All of these shampoos are extremely mild and will cleanse the hair without stripping it of vital moisture.

Don't be lured by "clarifying" shampoos that are made with intensive cleansers designed to remove the buildup from heavy styling products. By including dehydrating or abrasive detergents, such as sodium laurel sulfate, sodium lauryl sulfate, and cocoamphodiacetate, they strip the hair of both the buildup and the valuable nutrients and moisture, damaging the mane's protective layer. Another typically harsh shampoo category is dandruff-fighting formulas—these are very intense, and I don't recommend them for our fragile curly manes.

SHAMPOO HOW-TO

This sounds elementary, but shampooing is more than lather-rinse-repeat. I find that my new clients beat their hair to death—and I mean death—in the process of shampooing. They come to me, wondering why their hair splits, so I ask them to show me how they shampoo. They look at me awkwardly and say, "Shampoo, water, scrub, and rinse." Can you imagine what they're thinking? Then I have the nerve to take it a step further and say, "Go through the motions and show me." Now they're convinced I'm a pompous hairdresser and out of my mind. To pacify me—and you should see their facial expressions—they lift their hands to their head. Of course, I'm narrating from the background, saying, "Wet your hair with lukewarm water, and apply shampoo in your palm, not directly on your hair"—and already we are on two different tracks, as the client mimes pouring the bottle of shampoo straight onto her hair. I continue narrating my version: "Rub your palms together, and run your hands through your hair to distribute the shampoo. Then, using the cushions of your fingers, massage your scalp to remove oils." My client has gathered all of her hair on her head and is rubbing her flattened palms over her tresses—just as in a commercial! I go on: "Then, in a piano-playing effect, run your fingers downward to detangle and distribute the shampoo throughout the hair— to detangle as well as to cleanse." By now my client has all her hair piled up on top of her head, and she's scrubbing it to death while I shake my head in mock horror—then we simultaneously break into laughter and I explain myself.

Less is more with curly hair—the more you abuse it, the harder it is to control. The hair is very fragile, and the cuticle is always lifted off the hair shaft. By piling it up on top of your head and then rubbing it, you are breaking off the cuticle and causing a great deal of damage. Again, if you use light products, you don't need to scrub at all. So, off to get shampooed! Here are the steps:

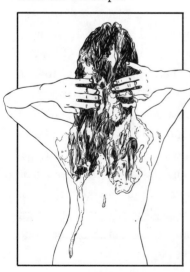

SIX-STEP SUDS UP
1. Saturate your tresses with warm water.
2. Place shampoo in your palm.
3. Rub your palms together, then run your hands through your hair to distribute the shampoo throughout your mane.

4. Using the cushions of your fingertips, rub the scalp only.

5. In a piano-playing motion, run your fingers downward to clean and detangle the hair. (Avoid piling tresses on top of your head while you shampoo—the more you scrub and tug, the more breakage you will get.)

6. Rinse with lukewarm water by separating your hair under the water instead of scrubbing.

CONDITIONING

Some people believe the hair and nails are dead, because they do not contain any nerves and do not feel pain when they are cut. Contrary to this belief, hair is a multistructured part of the anatomy and contains a cortex, medulla, and cuticle. My mantra is "Just as you must eat to survive, so must you feed your hair—to maintain its health, shine, and manageability." For this reason, I recommend nourishing the hair with a special deep conditioning treatment twice a month (or more) to restore its healthy pulse, which is regularly weakened by the environment and frequent styling.

What many people don't realize is that "instant conditioners" are different from nourishing hair treatments. Curly hair requires basic conditioning (with an instant or daily conditioner) after every shampoo, which serves to detangle fragile wet strands in order to create perfect curls without adding unnecessary stress. There are *no* lasting strengthening effects from any instant conditioner! The only way to truly feed your hair is via heated deep conditioners used on a regular basis. The ultimate path to beautiful hair—whether it has a light curl, medium curl, kinky curl, or mixed—is to deep-treat the hair. Feed it—it's the canvas of your painting, and without that foundation, there's no pretty picture. And believe me, I know, I've seen . . .

DAILY CONDITIONING HOW-TO

The key here is proper application. Never rub conditioner into your scalp. Keep the conditioner on the hair, not the skin, to allow the pores to stay clean and open to the air.

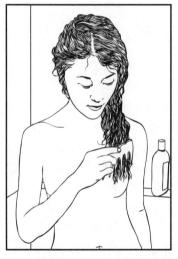

1. After shampooing, rinse your hair thoroughly with warm water by tilting your head back into the shower stream. If your hair is long, lean your head so that your tresses drape forward over one shoulder.
2. Pour a small amount of instant conditioner (one dime-sized dollop for short hair, one quarter for long hair) into the cupped fingers of one hand, then rub both sets of fingertips together. Begin applying conditioner two inches from your scalp by gathering your locks into a ponytail, and slide your hands down to the ends.
3. Using a piano-playing effect, run your fingers with conditioner on them through your hair to detangle and condition the hair shaft. Work it downward all the way to the end. Then use a wide-toothed comb from the bottom up. (*Note:* This is the last time you'll use a comb. After the shower, you'll only need to use your fingers.)

4. To rinse, separate your hair and run water through it without rubbing. The water will actually form your curls. Rub the scalp only with your fingertips to remove the conditioner, and allow your scalp to breathe.

5. Leave 25 percent of the conditioner on the ends for extra protection during the day. Your hair will feel slightly slippery at this point.

6. Never rub your hair with a towel to dry it—simply blot the excess water out to keep your curls set. Don't wrap your hair turban-style with a towel, either—you'll create a bend across the top of your head that will create frizz and distract the curl pattern.

AFTER THE SHOWER . . .

After your hair is rinsed, your curls are already set in place by the water. Simply drape a towel over your hair and gently blot out the excess water without disturbing your curl pattern. *Never* comb your hair—your fingers are your best tools!

MORE INCENTIVE TO FEED YOUR HEAD

By now you understand that curly hair is at a disadvantage— its corkscrew shape forces the outermost protective layer into a perpetually "lifted" position. As a result, this cuticle layer looks like ruffled feathers, leaving the internal, molecular layer exposed to dehydration. This core layer is where your hair color and overall condition are retained, so it's important to protect it.

The molecules themselves are made of elongated proteins that look like a chain of unpeeled peanuts. When these links are connected, the hair has the inner weight it needs to fall into healthy spirals and emit a healthy shine. The cuticle remains closed and smooth, which allows the hair shaft to retain vital moisture and nutrients. Locks respond better to styling and won't contract as much during the drying process, which cuts down on frizz in humid conditions. It also allows the color to stay longer and not fade as quickly unless you are a beach person.

If the links are broken from dehydration and damage, the inner layer loses its weight, preventing strands from forming perfect curls. Light also passes through these gaps, providing a dullness. At this point, the dehydrated cuticle acts like a dry sponge and absorbs too much moisture, causing the hair shaft to bulge, creating a halo of tiny, lifted hairs—aka frizz.

DEEP CONDITIONING—
PLEASE READ THIS TWICE!

You must deep-condition your hair twice a month. By restoring nutrients lost through everyday life, your hair will maintain its internal weight, and your curls will remain vibrant and bouncy. This eliminates the need for topical aids, such as non-breathable waxes, silicones, and oils to weigh it down and provide an artificial shine.

Nourishing treatments use heat to soften the hair's proteins and replenish the hair with vital nutrients lost to environmental aggressors such as wind, air conditioning, and blow-drying. Remember, the simple act of shampooing is also dehydrating because the warm water opens the cuticle, and the cleansers flow into the hair shaft and rinse out many of the nutrients. When you're finished washing your hair, the cuticle is parched, the same way your skin feels tight after cleansing it, so frequent conditioning should be an automatic part of your hair care regime.

When I refer to deep conditioning treatments, I do *not* mean moisture packs with fatty hydrating supplements or hot oil treatments. These simply lubricate the hair and make it look and feel a little softer and shinier. In the long run, these formulas create dullness and dehydration. Oil and water do not mix and will never be able to saturate the hair with moisture.

To truly condition the hair, the protein molecules in the cuticle need to melt and bond together using low heat and an appropriate formula. A deep treatment should always require heat—if you see one that doesn't, don't waste your time and money. Follow the steps below for a first-class feeding:

DEEP TREATMENTS FIVE-STEP HOW-TO
1. Begin with freshly washed hair using a gentle shampoo.
2. Prep the ends with a little daily conditioner.
3. Apply at least two ounces or more of the treatment to your hair, working it in section by section. To envision the amount of coverage you'll need to adequately saturate your locks, imagine soaking your hair in a bowl full of treatment— you'll need ample proteins to fill all those "empty links" in your hair shaft.

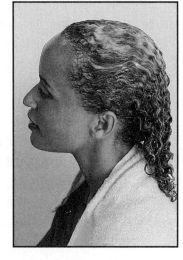

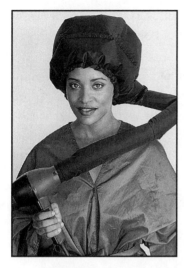

4. Cover your entire mane with a plastic cap, and apply heat using a hood-style dryer or bonnet attachment or a hand-held dryer to adequately warm your hair in about twenty minutes. (Allow extra time for very thick or long hair.) It's important to heat your hair thoroughly to relax the cuticle proteins and allow the absorption of key ingredients to reconnect the internal molecular layer, restoring its inner weight. Be sure to use low heat and maintain the level for the full twenty minutes in order for the heat to swell the hair shaft and for the proteins to penetrate it.

Alternative Heating Methods
* Wrap hair in a warm towel or heating pad.
* Sit in the sun or a sauna.
* Sleep with treatment in your hair overnight.
* *Note:* For those with thick or coarse hair, such as people of African or Middle Eastern heritage, you will not benefit from leaving the treatment in your hair overnight. Your body temperature alone will not be enough to heat the hair and soften the cuticle, and your hair may become tangled and matted. You must heat your hair thoroughly using one of the other methods.

5. After you've heated your hair, remove the plastic cap and apply an instant conditioner throughout the mane—on top of the deep treatment. Allow hair to cool for ten minutes, then rinse with warm-to-cool water, but do not shampoo.

   Now you're ready to style as usual, as recommended for your hair type. With the correct deep treatment, you can't overcondition your hair because it won't build up or weigh down your tresses.

   Allow the treatment to continue its work by waiting to shampoo for a few days.

ABOUT OUIDAD DEEP TREATMENT

This book came about not because I have a product line but because I was asked to write it in light of my success at working with curly hair. That said, I feel comfortable talking about my Deep Treatment, which is the cornerstone of my business. The Ouidad Deep Treatment is made up of a mixture of twenty-one amino acids, sulfides, citric acids, and antioxidants, and many different types of proteins. It's designed to help connect your molecular layer by relinking the chain reaction, allowing the hair to have its own internal life. Nothing is permanent—just as I said; your hair is in a corkscrew shape and your cuticle layer is lifted, so the hair is susceptible to losing its own internal layer (molecular layer) by environmental damage alone. Never mind what we do to it—blowing, coloring, straightening, perming, flat irons—ouch! Need I go on? I'll spare you—only because I don't know you that well. So that's why you need to condition every other week to help your hair stay healthier.

I've seen the Deep Treatment forgive a variety of sins—it

can strengthen damaged hair and keep healthy hair from getting damaged. But it can't repair hair that's "dead." For example, let's say your hair has been chemically straightened stick straight and is completely lifeless. Deep Treatment to the rescue. My elixir seeks out the salvageable strands and performs "hair CPR" on these limp locks, restoring them with a strong, healthy pulse. Of course it can't bring dead hair back from the grave—I refuse to promise the impossible. If hair is beyond help, I hate to say this dreadful line, but "Cut it and start all over again!"

Whether you use my Deep Treatment or another brand, the key to healthy hair is to feed it regularly with a protein-based formula. Check the Ingredients Guide in this chapter for specific names of hydrating proteins that you'll find on product labels. What you want to avoid are formulas featuring hot oils, emollients, and waxes—these are merely "feel good" products that give your mane a silky feeling but won't penetrate and nourish the hair shaft.

INGREDIENTS GUIDE

Shopping for hair care products is a dizzying experience. Each formula boasts a long list of benefits along with complicated and unfamiliar ingredients. I've made a list of what to look for to help simplify the selection process, whether you need shampoo, conditioner, or styling products or simply want to decode some of the high-tech language. Remember, the amount or percentage of any ingredient in a product always corresponds to the order in which it appears on the ingredients listing.

GOOD INGREDIENTS

Amino acids—These substances are used by the body to build the proteins that build the base of the hair; they are added to shampoos and conditioners to seal cracks in the hair shaft.

Ammonium lauryl sulfate—Typically found in shampoos and other cleansers, this substance provides essential moisture, reduces static, and increases pliability. It is derived from natural coconut alcohols. It is gentler than sodium lauryl sulfate, C14-16 olefin sulfate, sodium dodecyl sulfonate, or alkylbenzene sulfonate. (Many of these ingredients can strip the color from your hair.)

Antioxidants—These substances, found in vitamins, help repair and prevent cell damage caused by free radicals. Sources include ginkgo biloba, green tea, grapeseed extract, green algae (flavonoids), lycopene (beta-carotene), ginseng, licorice, rosemary, juniper, lipoic acids.

Castor oil (aka Palm Christi oil)—This seed extract is derived from castor bean plants; a great soothing, conditioning agent, it provides a smooth, shiny effect on hair; it is often used in styling gels.

Cetrimonium chloride (vegetable)—This substance is a cosmetic biocide, surfactant, and antistatic agent.

Cetyl alcohol (vegetable)—This vegetable-based, nondrying alcohol works as an emollient and a thickener.

Citric acids—Derived from citrus fruits, these substances are used as a preservative and pH balancer.

Cocamidopropyl betaine (aka coconut oil)—This substance provides essential moisture, reduces static, and increases pliability.

Dimethicone (quartz)—This water-soluble surface-active compound is derived from the mineral quartz; it reduces friction and static while holding moisture and adding softness and slip.

Disodium EDTA (mineral salt)—This chelating agent improves a product's performance in hard water.

DMDM hydantoin (preservative)—This substance is a broad-spectrum antibacterial preservative.

Emollient—This substance has moisturizing qualities.

Glycerin—This natural humectant is made of vegetable-based amino acids. It helps seal in moisture, keeps products from drying out the hair, and provides spreadability to products for even application.

Glyceryl stearate (corn)—This is an emollient conditioning agent.

Hydrolyzed castor oil—Derived from castor bean plants, this oil gives shine and moisture and helps seal the cuticle.

Hydrolyzed keratin—This protein is found in conditioners.

Hydrolyzed wheat protein—Derived from amino acid and enzyme, this substance helps to restore strength to hair.

Jojoba oil—Derived from the desert shrub *Simmondsia chinensis,* this oil is used as a lubricant and provides excellent conditioning qualities to hair and skin.

Olive oil—This oil provides excellent penetration into the hair shaft and gives sheen to the hair. It is used in hairdressing creams and/or shine agents.

Methylparaben (preservative)—This nonirritating, nonsensitizing preservative is colorless and odorless.

Mineral oil—One of the most benign of all cosmetic ingredients, this oil rivals water in terms of potential irritation.

Derived from earth minerals, it provides good conditioning for dry hair and slip for styling.

Panthenol/pro-vitamin B5—This vitamin moisturizes dehydrated sections and actually pumps the hair by attracting and holding in moisture. It also reduces static and increases pliability.

PEG-60 (almond glycerides)—This substance is an almond-based emollient.

pH—pH is not an ingredient but is the measure of acidity and alkalinity of a substance, on a scale of 1 to 10 (7 is neutral, below is acidic, above is alkaline).

Polyquaternium 11—This film former provides great combability, reduces static, detangles, and gives some thermal protection.

Retinyl palmitate (vitamin A)—This antioxidant vitamin is used for its moisturizing and conditioning properties.

Silicone—Silicone comes in many forms and is used in more than 80 percent of hair care products. Look for lightweight crystal silikats instead of greasy, plasticlike coatings. It gives an exquisite, silky feel because its components are related to fluid technology.

Silk amino acids—This protein, found in styling products, adds shine and body.

Sodium hyaluronate (bioengineered)—This substance acts as a net to hold moisture in and on hair while still allowing it to breathe.

Soy protein—This protein is found in conditioners.

Tocopheryl acetate (vitamin E)—This antioxidant vitamin is used for its healing and emollient properties; it conditions, moisturizes, and protects.

Wheat germ protein—This protein is found in conditioners.

Witch hazel extracts (*Hamamelis virginiana*/plant leaves, twigs, bark)—These extracts have astringent and soothing properties.

For conditioners, look for good detangling, conditioning, and softening agents, such as proteins, amino acids, elastin, wheat germ protein, soy protein, breathable panthenol, and quaternium.

BAD INGREDIENTS

Ammonium xylenesulfonate—This cleansing agent can be harsh to delicate hair. It is usually found in drugstore brands.

Balsam—Balsam is very astringent and can leave hair brittle. Some people may be sensitive to it; it can cause allergic reactions.

Camphor—As with balsam, this ingredient should not be applied to the skin or scalp, as it may cause dermatitis.

C14-16 olefin sulfate—This cleansing agent can be very harsh to delicate hair. It is usually found in drugstore brands.

Eucalyptus oil—Its antiseptic qualities can be drying to the hair and skin. Some people may be sensitive to it; it can cause allergic reactions.

Mineral clay—This clarifying agent is sometimes found in hair masks or conditioners. It can be very drying and damaging to the hair over time. It is best utilized for skin products only.

Sodium dodecyl sulfonate—This cleansing agent can be harsh to delicate hair. It is usually found in drugstore brands.

MYTH: *Too much protein will dry out your hair.*
TRUTH: Protein is often used to strengthen hair. Some proteins can make the hair stiff and lead to brittle, dry-feeling tresses. In actuality, these proteins are only giving hair the *feeling* of dryness. I counteract this problem by incorporating moisturizing wheat and soy proteins into my products—they add elasticity and give the hair a healthy "pulse."

MYTH: *All alcohol is damaging and drying to the hair.*
TRUTH: There are many varieties of alcohol—some for consumption, some for household use, and others for grooming. When choosing a product with alcohol, consider those with plant-derived alcohols, such as witch hazel, that act as liposolvents. This means they act like skin care products, moisturizing by emulsifying fatty acids and allowing other beneficial proteins to penetrate. While some alcohols are more dehydrating to the hair than others (such as SD alcohol and isopropyl alcohol), the important issue is the percentage of alcohol within a given product. Look for formulas with a low percentage—in other words, alcohol should fall at the end of the ingredients listing.

HOME REMEDIES

Aloe deep conditioner: Empty out the gel from leaves of an aloe vera plant. Combine this with equal parts of hydrolyzed milk to form a paste. Rinse well with water. The superconditioning amino acids from the aloe and milk provide shine and an excellent nourishing treatment.

Sunflower oil conditioner: Use this conditioning, breathable oil to help your hair hold in moisture. It's a great source of fatty acids, which help seal the cuticle and give each strand internal weight. Use enough oil to saturate your hair—for short hair, two tablespoons; for medium tight curls, one ounce; and for long tight curls, two ounces. Allow the oil to stay in your hair for twenty minutes, then shampoo and seal the cuticle with an instant detangling conditioner.

Yogurt masque: For a terrific curly hair masque, apply plain yogurt after a shampoo (skip the conditioner) to improve both bounce and shine. Use one tablespoon for medium-length hair and two tablespoons for shoulder-length or longer hair. Rinse well with water, and follow with a leave-in conditioner.

MYTH: *People with curly hair should use natural-bristle brushes.*

TRUTH: Curly hair should never be brushed! When wet, a brush may tear or stretch fragile strands, and when dry, it will separate and diffuse the curls, creating frizz. The best approach to styling curly hair is to detangle wet locks with a round-tipped, wide-toothed comb and position it with your fingers while still damp. The less contact your hands have with already-styled curls, the better! (The only exception to this rule is when straightening or smoothing curly hair, but this is not recommended for daily styling.)

TIPS
* Use leave-in conditioner on dry hair at the end of the day to give curls a wake-up call.
* Protect your tresses from the sun's dehydrating rays by applying a leave-in conditioner before you spend time outdoors.

* On humid days, add a deep conditioning treatment to your styling gel for extra hold and a frizz-free day.
* Always detangle your hair in the shower with a large-toothed comb while the conditioner is still in your hair.
* Detangle your hair from ends to roots to avoid knots and breakage.
* Never wrap a towel around your head turban-style because your hair will crease against its natural wave.
* If you wear your hair cropped short, shampoo daily.
* If you wear braids or extensions, be sure to cleanse the scalp thoroughly to keep the roots healthy to avoid breakage. To do this, spray a little leave-in conditioner on your braids—keeping them lubricated will avoid damage.

Style How-Tos

No matter what shape, size, and texture your curls are, my styling technique will produce healthy, defined tendrils. Here I've outlined the Ouidad Method for creating curls, plus other styling options based on your lifestyle needs.

Anecdote: One of the sweetest stories I know about curly hair concerns a bride-to-be who desperately wanted her curls to look perfect on her wedding day. Unfortunately, her wedding was scheduled far from the salon, and none of our staff could style her hair on her big day. I wanted to help, so I told her I would train one of her friends to do her hair. The bride arrived at the salon with none other than her groom! He patiently listened and watched as I demonstrated each step, then practiced the techniques until he felt comfortable. The bride knew he was the one person she could count on to make her happy!

THE OUIDAD METHOD:
STYLE CURLY

* Begin with wet hair, and gently squeeze out the excess water, using a towel to blot out additional moisture. Do not flip your head over or rub the hair briskly with the towel—

both methods will only fragment the curls and cause frizz. At this point, half your work is done.

* Using outstretched fingers, comb through a leave-in conditioning spray rich in vitamins and aloe vera to seal in the moisture. *Note:* As you condition and detangle, your goal is to keep the curls together and not fuss or shake your hair to avoid disturbing the waves.

* Rub a small amount of styling lotion between your palms, and smooth your hands over the hair in one fluid movement from front to back, as if you're gathering your hair into a ponytail. This move immediately delivers lotion to the hair's exterior to quickly control flyaway and baby hairs. Do this as soon as possible after showering for best results.

* From here, begin working dime-sized amounts of product into four sections of hair. (Create more sections for thick, unruly hair.) The first section will be the nape of the neck to the middle of the back of the head. The second section will start at

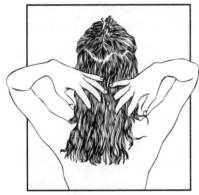

the back of the head and extend to the hairline. The last two sections will include the two sides. *No matter how thorough you think you are, you won't get complete coverage with one large application of styling lotion.*

* Rub the lotion between your palms, and work into

each section by combing your fingers through the hair from the scalp to the ends. As you apply, use your fingers to define each curl. Be *sure* to coat all of the hair in each section from roots to ends, to close the cuticle layer of the hair. Any strands left uncovered will become frizzy and throw off the even, "puzzle piece" flow of your curls.

∗ After raking your fingers through your hair from the scalp to the ends, don't let go of the ends right away. Hold on to them for a moment without actually pulling or overstretching the hair. Then gently shake the hair back and forth as you loosen your hold, to allow curls to form once again.

∗ Once you've applied your styling lotion, position your curls with duckbill clips.

∗ To break up any "crunchy" or stiff sections, take a finger full of pomade or glaze, and rub it between your palms until it melts. In one firm motion, smooth your hands over your entire mane (once it's dry) from front to back, as if you're creating a ponytail, then hold the ends for a moment and gently let go. With a little practice, you should be able to do this in a single gesture.

∗ Keep your curls in place with an all-over spritzing of light-hold styling mist (aka hairspray). This is also a perfect type of formula to spray on tresses as they dry, to encourage proper curl definition and hold. Anything stronger will become hard or gummy.

STRAIGHT STYLING

If you've reached this chapter, I hope you're learning to love your curls! But I also understand the curiosity and need for variety that prompts a desire to style your hair straight. As long as you feed your hair with frequent deep conditioning treatments, an occasional blow-drying session won't cause major damage. Bear in mind, the tighter the curl, the trickier the process. Here's how to go straight safely.

STRAIGHT TIPS

* Shampoo and condition before you blow-dry—never dry dirty hair. Curly hair will resist straight styling and simply break off. (*Tip:* Rinse the conditioner/detangler from your scalp, but leave a tiny bit on the ends to protect them from the blow-dryer.)

* Use a large round natural-bristle brush—plastic bristles will tear the hair's cuticle layer. Some people recommend paddle brushes, but I feel they don't provide the smoothness that a round brush offers. Use the largest-diameter brush you can hold comfortably— the larger the brush, the easier it is to smooth the hair.

* Spray a leave-in conditioner to restore the hair's elasticity and protect it from the dehydration and heat of the blow-dryer.

* Have several clips on hand to section the hair as you dry it. If you feel uncomfortable holding a brush in one hand and the dryer in the other, use a dryer with a brush attachment.

* Deep-condition the hair frequently if you blow-dry it straight regularly, to keep it moist and healthy.

STEP-BY-STEP BLOW-DRYING

BLOW-DRY CURLS ~ STRAIGHT

1. Divide clean, wet hair of medium length or longer into five sections: (1) the top, (2) and (3) the sides, (4) the crown, and (5) the nape. Secure each section with a clip.

2. Unclip the nape, and separate a one-inch section. Reclip the rest of the nape out of the way.

3. Place the brush at the roots, and let the bristles grip the hair. With your other hand, direct the dryer nozzle about two inches away from the hair, just above the brush and pointing downward.

4. Roll the brush down gently while the other hand follows with the dryer. Continue this motion all the way to the ends. (Trick: If you're right-handed, it's easier to hold the brush with your right hand and the dryer with your left.)

5. Repeat step #4 until the hair is completely dry. If you leave a hint of dampness in this type of hair, it will curl up immediately! When your hair is fully dry, it will have a glossy shine and no frizz.

6. Drying the hair section by section allows it to lie smooth and look shiny. The heat from the blow-dryer will force the cuticle layer to close and mold it straight with the help of the brush.

7. It should take about thirty to forty minutes to complete the entire head, working in the order I've suggested above. Finish by brushing your hair with the round natural-bristle brush, then rub a dollop of a finishing gel between your palms. Slide your hands on top of your head, gathering your hair into a ponytail and then

down to the ends. Hit the hair with the blow-dryer on the cool setting for extra glossy results. Give your mane a shake, and enjoy!

Tip: To maintain this look, simply tuck your hair into a shower cap when bathing and touch up with a blow-dryer. If you feel your hair is becoming greasy but don't want to restyle yet, dip a washcloth in witch hazel and run it through sections of your mane to freshen your look.

Anecdote: *"The day of my wedding, I had my long, curly hair blown straight at a salon. I was so happy that day, I danced up a storm. By the end of the evening, my hair took on a life of its own, transforming from smooth and straight to frizzy and huge! All the guests were staring at my hair, but I didn't understand why until I saw the photos. I still had a blast!"*

BLOW-DRY CURLS ~ WAVY

1. Blot clean, wet hair with a towel to a damp-dry state. Be gentle to avoid disturbing the curl pattern.
2. Apply a lightweight styling lotion as evenly as possible, and let it air-dry until it's 90 percent dry.
3. Grab three-inch sections of curls, and pull them downward to release their "grip," while hitting the hair with a blow-dryer with a diffuser attachment. This will soften the curls' hold and create a more relaxed curl pattern. Be careful—the harder you pull, the straighter your hair will get.

4. Do not section your hair with clips the way you would if you were blow-drying it completely straight—this will separate your curls and cause frizz. By handling various sections of hair, you'll wind up with long, smooth curls with lots of body.

5. Follow major blow-drying with plenty of deep conditioning. Feed! Feed! Feed!

Anecdote: *During my years of battling the straight hair magazines, I once did a personal survey. I took two models with the same hair color, one with straight hair, the other very curly. Both heads were healthy, shiny, and alive. I walked with them into a convention room. Both ladies attracted the same amount of attention.*

SET A MOOD

Many people assume curly hair has only two looks—loose and in a ponytail. Please! Curly hair is incredibly versatile. The key is positioning your curls correctly as they transition from wet to dry. Once you've mastered that art, you can do anything you want!

THE PROFESSIONAL LOOK

The number-one request I get at the salon is "Please make my hair look professional." Is that possible? Of course! A medium-length cut showcasing a combination of wavy and kinky curls in a crisp bob style is the perfect companion to a classic Chanel suit. Keep in mind that curly hair is multifaceted and can achieve many looks—and hold them much longer than straight hair. Curls are a frame of mind. No one can litigate a case, give a lecture, run a meeting, conduct a study, perform surgery, provide financial advice, report the news, or lead a country with hair unkempt and wild, whether it's straight, wavy, or curly. But with the perfect "carve and slice" cut and proper positioning of your curls, you can command professional attention and respect. Your hair will fall into smooth, even curls without the un-wanted puffiness and wild effect.

Anecdote: *"I graduated from Stanford University and landed an internship at a prestigious financial firm. My boss told me to*

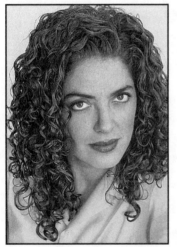

cut off my curls or he would not be able to hire me for full-time work—my hair did not fit the company's image."

Long, Sliced Bob: A great cut is the foundation for this easy, classic look. Simply follow the guidelines I've offered for styling curly hair. When your hair is dry, make sure to use my decrunching technique to eliminate the stiffness the gel

LONG, SLICED BOB

may leave: gather your hair in a ponytail shape, and run your flattened hands over your entire mane. Finish with a light-hold hairspray.

Slicked-Back Soft: Follow the directions for the Slicked-Back Bob, but run your fingers through your mane once it's dry to soften the look. Finish with a little hairspray.

Slicked-Back Bob: Towel-dry your clean, wet hair, then apply gel. Use a wide-toothed comb to create a shape—make a zigzag part, finger waves, whatever you want! Spray your tresses with a light hairspray, then dry completely with the diffuser.

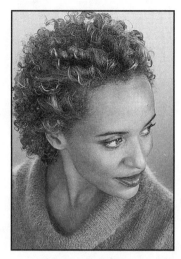

SLICKED-BACK BOB

Slicked-Back Twist: Follow the directions for the Slicked-Back Bob, except gather your hair in a neat French twist instead of leaving the ends loose.

Tools needed: wide-toothed comb, defrizzing gel, finishing pomade, light-hold hairspray, blow-dryer diffuser

Anecdote: *When I wear my shoulder-length hair in natural curls, my clients often comment on my "wild look," but when I slick my hair back, they call me "The Boss!"*

THE ROMANTIC LOOK

Curly hair has always been viewed as romantic—think of all the movies, plays, and myths that feature lovestruck, wavy-haired maidens. Romeo and Juliet, Adam and Eve, Rapunzel. These looks rarely waver: a mane of curls, coifed half up and half down, soft tendrils positioned throughout the hair, or curls pinned up and cascading off the scalp. Here's how to do it.

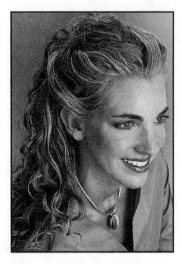

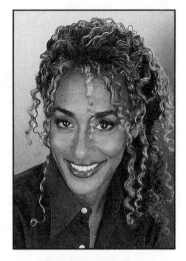

CASCADING UPDO   CASCADING PONY

Cascading Updo: Without destroying your curls, gather two to three tendrils and pin them up about three to four inches. On the sides, lift the hair and pin using the Crown of Curls technique. On the top of the head, the tendrils should be pulled back and pinned on a diagonal for security.

Cascading Pony: Hold your hair upside down, and gather it into a loose ponytail (using a scrunchie the same color as your mane), allowing the section at the nape to remain free. Choose a few sections within the ponytail to tighten with bobby pins—tuck the tips of the pins into your hair to hide them. This is a great look for thick, fine curls.

Crown of Curls: Dry your hair using the Ouidad Method so that there's no part and your locks are directed toward the back of your head. Slide your thumb and index finger over your ear, forming an inverted V, gathering a small section of hair. Without making your hair too taut, lift these tresses and place them in the rounded part of a bobby pin. Take the points of the pin and tuck them into other curls toward the back of your head. You want to hide the bobby pin, instead of sliding it across a flat section of hair. Repeat this technique on the other side. To soften the look, pull a few tendrils over your brows, or let some curls cascade over the parts you've pinned up.

Tools needed: blow-dryer diffuser, styling lotion, bobby pins, lightweight styling mist

THE SEXY LOOK

An absolutely gorgeous head of long shiny curls couldn't be any sexier, as we see on our favorite celebrities: Sarah Jessica Parker, Goldie Hawn, Julianna Margulies. Showcase your curls by letting them cascade past your shoulders.

Mix and Match: For a sexy, tousled effect, vary the size of your curls with the help of a curling iron. For loose and medium curls, use a medium-barrel iron, and for kinky curls, use a larger barrel. Although I generally discourage the use of curling irons, you can safely use one if it's covered with a tissue or handkerchief. This extra protective layer works the way a muslin cloth does when you are ironing silk fabric. Separate the hair into small sections, and loosely wrap (don't twist) the hair *from the roots to the ends.* Leave the hair on the barrel for a few seconds, then slide the iron out. Allow the hair to cool, and use your fingers only to gently position your curls. For extra staying power on loose curls, spray your locks with a light hairspray before using the curling iron.

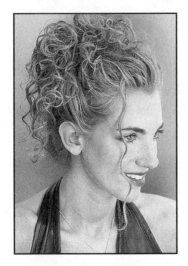

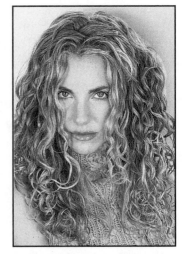

UNDONE UPDO   **SEX KITTEN COIF**

Undone Updo: Gather three-quarters of your hair, twist it into a loose bun, and secure it with a decorative chopstick. Be sure to let the "tails" stick out, and allow any loose tendrils to fall naturally. This is a great look for long, kinky curls. You can substitute a handful of bobby pins for the chopstick. Just gather sections of curls and secure at the nape until you've pulled back three-quarters of your hair. Crisscross the bobby pins for extra hold.

Sex Kitten Coif: Wear your hair loose and natural, but as you diffuse-dry it, gently pull on each tendril to soften and loosen your curls. Your hair is sexiest in its natural state!

THE FUN LOOK

Short curls, combed while wet to create a half-curl-half-wave style, are both playful and easy. Another quick look is to slick it all back, while your tresses are wet, with lots of styling gel and a misting of hairspray.

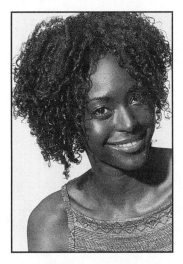 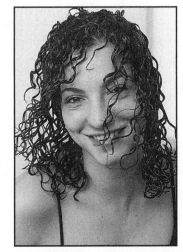

CARNIVAL OF CURLS   **SLICK CURLS**

Carnival of Curls: Create a youthful, crazy look by letting your hair dry naturally (coat in defrizzing gel first), and allow your curls to expand. Enjoy their bounce and body!

Slick Curls: Apply a generous dose of styling gel to the hair for a wet effect, but don't comb it smooth. Allow your natural curl pattern to shine through.

Combo Curls: While your hair is still wet, comb the top half into finger waves and allow the lower half to dry curly. Saturate the hair with gel before shaping it. Use clips to hold the waves and diffuse the entire head. It's a popular look on the runway right now.

Roller Derby: For an ultrafunky set, part your hair in the middle and use Velcro rollers (small for fine/kinky and loose curls; medium for small/tight curls). Start with wet hair coated with gel, then use a roller (rolled under) on alternating layers of hair. Diffuse-dry the whole head, and finish with a light hairspray.

Tools needed: Blow-dryer diffuser, gel, Velcro rollers, hairspray, duckbill clips

ACCESSORIES

Many of my clients yearn to wear trendy little hair clips and headbands, but they get frustrated when they try to position them. To avoid funny cowlicks and "antennas," insert your accessories with the natural flow of your curls. Don't pull a section of hair tight against your head and try to secure a barrette—you'll wind up with a bulky section just beyond the clip. Also, don't overstuff a barrette, or you'll get a similar problem. As for headbands, stick to thin wire ones for invisible hold instead of the wider versions that will disrupt your curl pattern. Your best bets are decorative chopsticks, bobby pins, and wide-toothed combs. These allow you to position your hair in different styles without crushing your curls.

MORE COIFS AND CURL CUES

Twist and Shout: Try this trendy knotted effect for daytime. Apply a defrizzing gel to your mane, then create a middle or side part. Pull your hair tight, and make a ponytail to one side. Twist the ends into a knot, securing with hairpins and adding more gel for extra hold. Repeat these steps on the other side, and let the back sections remain hanging loose.

Twisted Mini Braids: Prepare for an evening out by applying a deep conditioning treatment to your wet hair and dividing the hair into five small braids. Let your tresses dry naturally, then secure the ends with a decorative accessory. The hair will dry looking sleek and shiny.

Casual Friday Ponytail: Allow your hair to dry in its natural curl pattern with some leave-in conditioner. Gather your hair to one side in a messy ponytail, allowing several tendrils to escape. Apply styling lotion to these pieces for extra control. At the end of the day, for a night on the town, pull more tendrils out of the ponytail and give them a twirl with some styling lotion.

Sea Set: Next time you're at the beach, apply a deep conditioning treatment to your wet hair. Divide your mane into five sections from front to back, then twist each section to the rear of your head. Gather all five sections in a ponytail, and allow your hair to dry this way throughout the day. When you get home, gently unwind the twists for a wavy, fun effect.

Sun Soother: Before you spend a day outdoors, leave in your daily conditioner (or soak your locks in a deep conditioner) to help control the frizzies and protect your tresses from the sun. While you enjoy the sand and surf, the sun's warmth will activate the conditioner and feed your hair.

Pool Cues: After swimming in chlorine, rinse your tresses immediately with water, and use a daily conditioner to help rebalance the minerals in your hair.

Bed Head Rx: To banish bed head without shampooing, wet down your hair with a leave-in conditioning spray, and restyle your curls with a little gel.

Hat Head Defense: Prevent your winter hat from squashing your curls by rolling a few tendrils into pincurls held loosely with bobby pins. When you come inside, you can quickly remove the pins, and your curls will look fresh and springy.

Curly to Wavy Tip: To create waves from tighter curls, take sections of almost-dry hair, and twist them into buns all over your head. Hit them with a warm hair-dryer, then allow them to cool. You'll discover soft, gentle waves when you let down the buns.

Extra Advice: I strongly advise against curling irons. They can singe the hair and destroy the cuticle (the outer, protective layer of the hair). If you must use a curling iron, be sure that your hair is completely dry first. Using a curling iron on wet hair can quickly bring the moisture in the hair to the boiling point, causing damage and breakage.

A request: When using bobby pins, I beg you to choose ones that match your hair color!

Anecdote: *"As an actor, I am often faced with hours of shooting the same scene over and over. My patience can handle this, but my curly hair cannot. With time, my hair becomes bigger and bigger. I always pray for a quick shoot—I'm afraid my puffy hair will cost me a job."*

Finishing Touches

At this point, you've learned how to care for and style your curls. This chapter focuses on the final stages of styling that can make or break your look. Even a healthy head of hair can go haywire with the wrong gel or improper drying technique. Remember, you're only as good as your tools!

THE RIGHT WAY TO USE A BLOW-DRYER

When used correctly, your blow-dryer can be a friend instead of a weapon. Delicate curls do not benefit from blasts of intense heat, so select a dryer with several heat settings, and pretend the highest levels don't exist.

Using a blow-dryer without a diffuser will spoil natural curls. Diffusers provide indirect air flow that won't dilute or flatten your waves. For best results, apply your styling products, then jump-start the process with some fairly direct heat on the key sections around your face. This will encourage the hair to dry in the desired style. Allow the rest of your hair to dry for ten to fifteen minutes before diffuse-drying your locks on a low setting from underneath (to prevent flyaways). Hold the hair gently and away from your scalp, focusing the heat on the roots. There's no need to "scrunch" the hair—that technique will separate your curls. To loosen your curls while you're diffusing, hold individual curls by the ends and gently tug downward while directing the blow-dryer on them.

After your hair is dry, it will have a "crunchy" feel if you've applied your styling lotion correctly. For softer curls that have motion and bounce, use my special maneuver: Gather all the hair as if you were making a ponytail, running your palms along the shape of your head and then down over the length of your hair. After a few tries, you'll be able to do this in one fluid motion. It will eliminate the stiff, crusty feeling without sacrificing your curls. For long hair, try gathering the hair in a few sections. To further soften your waves, you may want to try this trick with a bit of pomade or finishing glaze in your palms.

STEAM HEAT

Dry heat is the product of a blow-dryer, air conditioner, or electric indoor heating. Steam heat, on the other hand, is moist and is found in the shower, under a bonnet hair-dryer, or inside a shower cap. Unlike dry heat, steam heat warms and softens the proteins in the hair. This is terrific for deep conditioning but horrible for styling. It's comparable to styling your hair on a rainy, humid day.

STREAMLINING YOUR HAIR CARE ARSENAL

Many of us are guilty of purchasing dozens of hair care products that we never use and that simply gather dust in the bathroom. In most cases, people are selecting formulas that are inappropriate for their hair type, or they are using the products incorrectly. Curly hair requires a certain number of must-have products as well as a set of must-nots. Stick to good, breathable formulas that won't suffocate your hair—they serve as a reminder to retain your curl pattern. So do yourself and your family a favor and eliminate the other products from your curly hair collection.

Anecdote: Once people understand—and love—their curls, they seem to see life differently. One client told me she has more time to spend with her kids because she's not wasting hours every week with the blow-dryer. Another woman claims that traveling is easier now that she wears her hair curly—she has no need to lug an extra suitcase filled with curling and flat irons, hot rollers, brushes, and three kinds of gel! After years of struggling to detangle her daughter's curls, a new client credits our Botanical Boost with improving their relationship! One woman wrote to me that her boyfriend was always frustrated when he tried to run his fingers through her kinky curls. After she visited me a few times and learned how to handle her curls, her frustrated boyfriend is now her loving fiancé! What I hear most often from new clients is that their confidence increases as they learn to work with their curls instead of fighting them. People also notice and admire a healthy head of curls, which does wonders for self-esteem.

SAY GOOD-BYE TO:

* ⋆ THICKENING OR VOLUMIZING SHAMPOOS, CONDITIONERS, AND STYLING AIDS: Curls thrive on definition, not volume. A curl's natural personality already provides enough body to eliminate the need for mane-boosting formulas like these.
* ⋆ HAIRBRUSHES: As previously mentioned, bristles are too harsh for fragile curly strands when they're wet, and will separate already-coifed curls.

* ALCOHOL-BASED PRODUCTS: Not only are curls delicate, but they are typically dry, which means that dehydrating alcohol-based formulas will only encourage unruly, frizzy tresses.
* MOUSSE: This styling foam is primarily used for adding volume to hair—a low priority for curls, which provide it naturally. Mousse is also tough to distribute evenly because it dehydrates almost before you can apply it.
* THICK/"EXTRA HOLD" GELS: These sticky concoctions are also difficult to apply evenly throughout your mane, creating imbalanced levels of hold. Curls thrive on a smooth, thin layer of styling product for a long-wearing, fluid look.

MYTH: *Curly hair requires thick, heavy styling products to prevent frizziness.*
TRUTH: Because curly manes are typically fine and delicate, heavy products will only dull and weigh down your strands, masking the beauty and body of your curls. Lightweight stylers, such as lotion, pomade, and glaze, provide hold and moldability without stifling the spring of natural curls.

MYTH: *Mousse is the best styling product for curly hair.*
TRUTH: Pack those cans of mousse along with your leg warmers and shoulder pads into a 1980s time capsule. Styling foams are both outdated and inappropriate for curly hair. Mousse adds volume to the mane—typically the last thing someone with curly hair needs. Mousse is also notorious for dehydrating the hair, another no-no when choosing products for curly hair. Curls look best when styled with lightweight

lotions that allow hair to fall into its own natural curl pattern, not with sticky mousses and gels that force it into place.

SILICONE AND PETROCHEMICALS, THE SILENT KILLERS

While environmental abuses to hair cause dryness and add to curly hair's fragility, suffocating styling products are equally damaging. Products containing waxes, oils, animal fats, and silicones from petrochemicals have been developed to add manageability to hair. While these ingredients were initially used in styling aids, they soon found their way into our daily regimen, including cleansing, conditioning, and stylers. When these ingredients are used in moderation, the hair is not at severe risk. But constant use is counterproductive to healthy hair.

Your hair is inherently reactive to climatic changes—it actually breathes and has a "pulse." Just like the rest of your body, it needs to breathe for survival. When it is suffocated beneath layers of hair products, it becomes dehydrated and malnourished and, as a result, dry, brittle, and frizzy. If you've ever worn fake nails, you know what happens to the natural nails beneath—they wither. Your hair reacts the same way under stifling substances, because hair and nails are both made of proteins called keratin.

Low-quality, thick serums coat the hair shaft, preventing strands from breathing. Once curls are suffocated and weighed down by the formulas, they cannot spring into healthy, defined waves and are impervious to other nourishment.

THE EXCEPTION: Silicone made from crystalline quartz is a breathable, water-soluble form that rinses easily from the hair without the use of a harsh, detergent shampoo. Look for it as "crystal silikat" on product labels.

Anecdote: *My clients turn into freelance publicists for me! One woman is such a loyal Ouidad fan, she claims to offer styling tips in ladies' rooms and haircut suggestions on the New York subways. It's like being in love—once you feel good about your hair, you want everyone to feel good too.*

STYLER SHOPPING LIST

* **MOISTURIZING FORMULAS**—These conditioning products hydrate parched locks to prevent and hide dryness, frizz, and damage. Look for breathable ingredients such as plant extract oils and vegetable-based proteins. Steer clear of oils and silicones, which will only weigh down and choke curls.

* **STYLERS DESIGNED FOR CURLS**—Many companies have created products to enhance and protect natural curls.

* **LIGHTWEIGHT LOTIONS**—Don't weigh down fragile tresses with thick, stifling gels and creams. Instead, saturate damp strands with liquidlike styling lotions to position curls.

* **FINISHING GLAZE**—Seal in moisture and avoid frizz with a quick coating of this thin syrupy formula.

* **POMADE**—This styler feels like heavy Jell-O or a light Vaseline. Used in small amounts, it's a great finishing product for smoothing out fine baby hairs and providing luster. This is the product to use to eliminate that "crunchy" effect from styling gel once your hair has dried. Rub the pomade between your hands, and run your palms over your hair as if gathering it into a ponytail. This single motion should soften the exterior yet leave the hold untouched.

* LIGHT HAIRSPRAY—A mild hairspray or styling mist is very important (and often forgotten) in preventing frizz.
* BALMS/WAXES—I consider these products "hair toys"—they're great for experimenting with shapes and special effects but not designed for serious hold or curl retention. These heavy formulas will weigh down your curls, so use them for more streamlined looks. *Note:* Do *not* use wax or silicone on colored hair—either one will interfere with your color.
* DUCKBILL CLIPS—These long metal clips, often used to hold rollers in place, are used to position wet hair. Remember, how your hair looks when it's dry depends greatly on what you do with it when it's wet. The hair's shape and style can be influenced or encouraged by positioning the roots at the moment it begins to dry. Use the duckbill clips to direct your curls, create height, and keep hair off the face. The trick is to slide the clips in standing on edge, not flat, for the most natural look.
* DIFFUSER—A simple hair-dryer is not compatible with curly hair because its nozzle directs too much air at each curl, deflating its volume and shape. Invest in a diffuser attachment to provide a steady source of heat without the pressure of a standard nozzle. Each wave will remain formed and maintain its natural body.
* WIDE-TOOTHED COMB—Hairbrushes are a curl's worst enemy—the multitude of sharp bristles can tear wet strands. So do your detangling with a comb. Neither comb nor brush should touch already-styled curls—this will only promote frizz and separate carefully defined tendrils.

ABOUT POMADE AND GLAZE

Your type of hair will dictate whether you use pomade or glaze. If your hair is frizzy and superfine, you may need to use both, by combining pomade with a styling lotion and following with glaze to finish the hair and break up the curls. Pomades typically have extra humectants to moisturize and soften the hair, making it a good choice for coarse, thick, dry, or unruly hair. A glaze is lighter and works well on medium to fine textures that are neither kinky nor dry.

HOW TO APPLY YOUR STYLING PRODUCTS

Your fingers are your best application tools. Use them to distribute lotions and gels in sections. How large or small you make each section will determine the size of your curls. But less is more with curly hair—the less you play with your curls, the easier they are to style, so let your fingers do their job, and then hands off!

LOGICAL LOCKS—MORE ADVICE ON STYLING

One of my clients told me she was frustrated because her hair wouldn't stay in the position she created when it was wet. She said she followed all my styling steps—and then went out and weeded her garden! I was flattered that she thought my products and advice were more powerful than *gravity*! Hairstyling is a logical, not a magical, process. You need to help your hair keep its style as it dries by holding your head upright. I'm not suggesting sitting perfectly still for hours, but steer clear of the garden, scrubbing the floors, or exercise class until your hair has a chance to dry.

Anecdote: *One of my clients visited me this summer before going on a cruise in Italy. I warned her of the tremendous humidity and suggested she slick back her hair with gel to make her life easier. She had other ideas. She thought she'd indulge in the services of the ship's salon and have her hair done—only to end up looking like the bride of Frankenstein. The stylist didn't even own a diffuser—she had to borrow my client's! She rubbed this poor woman's hair with a towel and then used every product and tool in the salon until she looked like she'd stuck her finger in an electric socket. After a bout of crying, she wisely washed her hair and reached for the gel—and spent the rest of the cruise enjoying herself!*

The Perfect Hair

FINDING THE RIGHT STYLE

The first step to accepting and enjoying your curls is to get the right haircut. It's essential to choose a style that complements your hair's texture, so I've suggested several cuts that accommodate various types of curls.

Anecdote: "At sixteen years old my hair was very curly and big. My mom and I used to spend two hours every night controlling my hair so I could go to school the next day. I could never go out with my friends—all I ever did was work on my hair. I used to cry all the time and felt that I never looked good. Forget about a boyfriend. My middle and high school years were hell, until my senior year when my friend told me about you. I saved up and came to you for my senior prom. After you conditioned, cut, highlighted, and styled my hair, I looked great and felt great! At the prom, everyone admired my curls, and I was first runner-up to the prom queen. Thank you! Thank you! Thank you!"
Rachel L., Long Island, New York

Warning: I use the term *layers* to refer to different lengths of hair that have been "sliced" to reduce the weight and bulk of the curl. I do *not* use the term to refer to blunt cut sections that cause curls to shrink and bunch up at the ears and forehead!

THE RIGHT HAIRCUT FOR YOUR HAIR TEXTURE

*LOOSE: This is the most flexible hair texture—you can wear almost any style and length. Your hair loves staying curly, but it can also tolerate straight looks. As long as you have a decent "carving and slicing" haircut, you can wear a shag, a bob, and even bangs. Shorter, face-framing sections around the face will fall into fairly smooth pieces because loose curls will not support well-formed curls at these lengths.

*CURLY: The key with medium curls is to wear your hair long enough to stretch your curls so that they fall a little looser. If your hair is cut too short, the curls will shrink up and look tight. Your shortest sections should reach midneck length— and don't even think about bangs! Shoulder length or longer is ideal for this hair texture. A good test is to stretch a tendril from your forehead toward your chin. If the piece isn't long enough to reach your upper lip, your hair is too short! What most actresses with this hair texture do is create long, sliced layers that allow them lots of versatility. The length allows them to pull their hair up or back and gives it enough weight to form perfect curls when worn loose.

*KINKY: With this hair texture, you may be of African, Hispanic, or Middle Eastern descent. While you might be tempted to pull back your delicate baby-fine curls into a ponytail every day, resist the urge! That would cause incredible breakage. Instead, opt for a longer length that reaches your chin when dry and touches the center of your back when wet, or consider a supershort cut and spice it up with hair color.

MYTH: *A good haircut can prevent the frizzies.*
TRUTH: A cut works with the shape of the hair. Frizz is linked to the structure of the hair. A combination of deep conditioning treatments every two weeks and a good "carving and slicing" haircut will allow your curls to fall more naturally and closer to the scalp with much more freedom and movement.

AN INTRODUCTION TO CURLY HAIR

Like many of you, I have endured countless hours of frustration—even tears—after bad haircuts. The recurrent problem was what I called the Pyramid Effect, in which my hair would lie limp at the roots and then puff out at the ends into a mass of frizz. In 1975 I finally took matters into my own hands and began experimenting with different cutting techniques. I created a unique method called "carving and slicing," which provides a more even, natural effect and reduces the unwanted volume without ruining the curls. Carving and slicing encourages the curls to fall into a "puzzle reaction," in which each spiral fits into the next, creating a smooth, even pattern. Once your hair is unburdened by flattening unruly layers, styling will be much easier.

I am in the process of training salons around the country to use the carving and slicing technique, so that clients can go to a local stylist for a professional curly haircut. Until then, look for stylists who use a vertical cutting motion that literally chisels out small sections of hair to reduce the weight of heavy clumps of curls, allowing strands to fall into perfect, defined spirals instead of larger, shapeless, overwhelming layers. *Slicing* is most effective on medium to fine manes. *Carving* is used most frequently on very fine hair, encouraging a larger curl pattern instead of many smaller, uncontrollable curls. Both methods allow the hair to sit closer to the scalp, thus creating a more relaxed, natural style for any mane.

The bottom line: A great haircut is the foundation to managing curly hair. In the past twenty-six years of magic making with curly hair, I've discovered I'm nowhere if I don't have this essential foundation. It's a losing battle without the proper framework!

CARVING AND SLICING VERSUS LAYERING, TEXTURIZING, AND THINNING

I'll be blunt. If your stylist suggests "layering," "texturizing," or "thinning" your hair, run from the salon and don't look back! These are three of the worst methods for cutting curly hair. *Layering* creates horizontal, shelflike blunt cuts throughout your mane. The shorter layers shrink up into fat sausage-like rolls, forming the dreaded Earmuff Effect. Unless you're attending a costume party as Princess Leia, avoid layered cuts. (When I refer to "layers" in this book, I am talking only about different lengths of hair, not these thick ledges of hair that cause so much grief.) *Texturizing* has become a catchphrase in the salon world, but it is best left to our straight-haired friends. The process involves snipping random pieces of hair to redefine the shape and add dimension to the hair. On curls, these missing sections of hair cause unevenness, unwanted shrinkage, and frizz because the balance of each wave is thrown off. Straight hair benefits from these texturized bits here and there to create a multidimensional effect that we curly girls possess naturally. Bottom line: Those seemingly aggravating "nuances" that our curls create are coveted by people with flat locks. *Thinning shears* are an antiquated tool that look like scissors with tiny combs attached. The shears cut exactly one half of the chosen section of hair, so one half shrinks up into a tight curl and the other half remains long and limp. Not a great combination!

Anecdote: This story is one of my favorites. After fighting with her curly hair for over forty years, a Detroit woman was given a special fiftieth birthday gift from her sister—a haircut with me! She had been reading about my curly hair techniques for years and had dreamed about coming to New York for a fabulous haircut. In order to make the trip, she saved her money and vacation time for two years! She worked in a car factory and couldn't afford a plane ticket, so she and her sister decided to drive by motorcycle to New York. They contacted the Harley-Davidson association, which gave them a route to follow and provided places to stay along the way. It also helped the ladies find safe parking in New Jersey and gave them instructions on riding the bus into Manhattan for the big day. She told me all of Detroit knew she was coming to the salon! In her letter to me, she said, "The money and physical exhaustion it took to get to your beautiful salon were worth it! You treated me like a queen, and you educated me, so now my hair always looks great. You were extremely generous when you gave me your products—and even today, three months later, I can still do my hair the way you taught me. I'll definitely see you again! Thank you. P.S.: I've enclosed a picture of my curls and my bike— my two most prized possessions!"

Jane from Detroit

FINDING THE PERFECT HAIRSTYLIST

For curly-haired people, a good stylist is essential to managing our manes. Because living with curls requires a few tips and tricks, we often think we have a better understanding of curly hair than many stylists. Admit it—you've even tried to cut your own hair because you have a sense of where and where not to snip. However talented you are, I don't recommend cutting your own hair. Curls are tricky—leave cutting them to the pros. The real talent is finding the right stylist! Here's how.

Word of mouth is the best form of recommendation when shopping for a great haircut. Ask people who have your hair type where they get their hair cut. Most of my clients come to me as referrals. I cut one woman's hair and she likes it, so she tells her friends, and they come to me and recommend me to more people. It snowballs quickly!

While you're researching stylists, *ask how long he or she has been in the business* and *use your intuition* when you meet. If it's someone you feel comfortable with, you'll probably get a great haircut and return for another. When we find someone good, we stick with them for a long time. When I first met one of my clients, we clicked immediately and got into such a deep conversation, she began to cry! She's been a loyal client ever since.

Another approach is to *choose a salon by its reputation* and *ask for someone who works with your specific hair type*. It's also important to *determine ahead of time what you want from your stylist*. If you're looking for trendy and sophisticated, then find a stylist who looks the part. That usually means they "believe" in that style and have the ability and interest to take you there.

When you meet that stylist, don't simply surrender! Make

your experience a partnership. Many first-time clients say to me, "You're the master. You know best." Although I'm flattered, I also can't read minds. I see you from the outside, and I certainly don't go home with you and take care of your hair. As a stylist, I enjoy cutting hair when my client and I understand each other and have the same goal. What I don't enjoy is a client who practically holds the scissors for me. I need some freedom to create—no stylist can work when he or she is stifled—but we all appreciate a mutual direction. Once I get to know a client, I earn her trust. She winds up getting a lot more out of me when she says, "Do whatever you want!" I love being free, and most clients allow this unless they have a specific fantasy style they're willing to take me through. Once we're both comfortable, believe me, I'll be happy to take charge!

Getting a haircut and finding a stylist is an important undertaking. Not only are you paying hard-earned money, but you are submitting yourself to a service that will affect you for the next two to three months. So be smart and do your homework before your appointment.

Once in a while, I get a client who comes in with a magazine clipping. Almost 90 percent of the time, the style doesn't fit her hair type. So I tease her—especially my beloved client Carol. It's become a habit over the past fifteen years. My reaction is to send her home with "homework." "Bring me several photos, each one describing a different section of your hair and hair type, and from these pictures, make a complete style." I know what to do with Carol's hair, but this way, she's forced to really think about her hair and understand it. Whenever I do this with a client, it happens only once! Don't get me wrong—I'm not discouraging photos, I'm explaining how I use them.

Another important factor in this relationship is to *be honest with your stylist.* Confess all your committed crimes—the colors, the straighteners, the blow-dryer abuse, and your conditioning schedule. I love it when a client conveniently forgets all she has done, and I stand behind her and say, "All right. Confess!" Inevitably, she turns red with embarrassment, and we both burst out laughing.

More advice: Please don't sit in the chair and tell your stylist who else has cut your hair. It's unnecessary information and can intimidate or offend your stylist. Remember, if you two click, this could be a long-term relationship, so you'll want to maintain a positive attitude. I have clients who have been with me for sixteen to twenty years, and every time I see them, they find a way to mention our years together. I'm proud to hear it and lucky! I haven't taken on any new clients for three and a half years!

Anecdote: I just met a woman in the salon who was clutching a tattered magazine clipping of a model with beautiful curls. She was desperate for this haircut, but every stylist she met told her it wasn't possible. When we met, I felt this look could work for her. She was so happy, she kept stopping other people in the salon and saying, "Do you know how long I've been carrying around this picture? Finally, there's someone who can do my hair the way I want it!"

BUILDING A RELATIONSHIP WITH YOUR STYLIST

THE CONSULTATION
If this is your first meeting, a consultation should take place in which you establish a mutual understanding of what is going

to happen to your hair. Your main objective is to determine your comfort level with this stylist. Here's what should be covered:

1. Your lifestyle, not your personal business
2. How much time you spend on your hair after every shampoo
3. How often you shampoo
4. Your weaknesses with your hair
5. How short or different you'd like to go
6. If you should start on a gradual plan for your hair or go for the ultimate cut right away
7. Your likes and dislikes about your hair

WHAT TO ASK YOUR STYLIST
1. What texture is my hair?
2. How much of a trim do I need?
3. What are my options with my type of curls?
4. Can I wear my hair either straight or curly with this cut?
5. What are my length options?
6. How often should I see you for a trim?
7. How much time will I need to spend on styling?

Now that you know how to find a stylist and work with him or her, it's time to switch gears. Love them and leave them! It happens to the best of us. Over the years I've gotten busier and busier and more and more popular. It became hard to see all my clients and give them the attention they were used to. During a difficult two-year period, I had to adjust to my new "stardom," and my clients had to adjust to my dwindling time with them. It was hard on all of us.

One client resolved the whole situation, and I cherish her for it. She took me aside and said she'd been watching my popularity grow for the past several years and was so happy for me. Unfortunately, she was a very needy person, and I was having a hard time fulfilling her needs. Who would I recommend from my staff to satisfy her? That was one of my most important life lessons: I immediately looked at what I was doing and referred many clients to my staff. I cut back on the number of clients I saw so that I could provide the ones I did see with the individual attention they deserved.

So tell your stylist you need a change or that you are trying someone new. Don't leave on a sour note—you want to be sure you can return on good terms.

MY ULTIMATE HAIR STORY

Believe it or not, I too was a hair victim. Despite my strong personality, I felt my curls controlled me. For years my thick curly hair suffered mercilessly with the Earmuff Effect, two-level pyramids, and styles that looked as if the top section of my hair were about to take off with me.

We all have an ultimate hair story—here's mine. I was twenty-two years old and had just arrived in New York City. I was invited to a Halloween party at Studio 54 with my friends with whom I worked in the theater doing hair and makeup. For the party, we were told to dress up as famous actresses, so I chose Joan Crawford, in her famous shot "The Fitting." The look was extreme: garter belt and nylons, padded shoulders, and a mink coat covering it all. The crowning glory was my head of hair teased and coaxed into the two large rolls Joan was famous for. It took some muscle to wrestle all my hair into the biggest, knotted, teased rolls you've ever seen, but it was Halloween, and I looked fabulous! The scary part came the next morning when I began unraveling my hair. What was I thinking? It took several of my friends and me half the day to detangle my teased hair. Imagine unwinding tight corkscrew curls that had been back-combed into each other. Talk about a fright! Half of my hair broke off in random places, leaving me with a "finger in the socket" effect. Phyllis Diller's crazy mane would have looked tame compared to mine.

My solution? I slicked back my hair for two weeks straight with a deep conditioning treatment in an attempt to help my hair externally and me internally! When I finally rinsed my hair, I discovered an erratic, multileveled array of springy curls. Fortunately, it was the 1970s and this wild look fit right in, just as it might today. Eventually, I had to face the scissors to give my curls the chance to repuzzle themselves together again. I've never attempted such a damaging style again, although I've experimented with different looks. Not surprisingly, my favorite look is short and simple!

Anecdote: "This is a must-share: My boyfriend and I were driving to meet his parents. It was a beautiful day, so we opened the windows, blasted the music, and sang all the way. When we arrived, his parents looked shocked. My hair was so big and windblown, it was horrible! I actually apologized for my hair!"

STRAIGHTENING, SOFTENING, SMOOTHING, RELAXING, PERMING: ONE PROCESS, MANY ERAS

If you've read this far, you now have a feel for my personality: I'm a passionate woman about life, and I'm very passionate about hair. As I said earlier, the reason I'm here today is to make sure no one will suffer any lack of self-confidence because of their curly hair. This has been my personal crusade! So when I see a client walk into my salon with gorgeous curls at the roots and stick-straight stiff ends, my first instinct is to jump up and down and say "Why? Why? Why? No more!"

I hope this book will encourage you to love your curls and show them off. I know the allure of smoother locks and chemical straightening treatments. But before you embark on a straightening endeavor, let me offer some information about it and provide tips to protect your mane.

First of all, the process of straightening hair goes by many names coined in different decades. *Softening, smoothing, relaxing, perming*—the process remains the same, with some variations of chemical formulas and strengths. What exactly is involved? Mainly a salon service, straightening requires a special chemical called sodium hydroxide to smooth out unruly strands. Depending on the strength of the chemicals, you can transform curly hair into softer waves or go completely straight. Before you begin this process, consult with your regular stylist to make sure your specific hair condition can endure the level of straightening you'd like. A good stylist will do a "strand test" to determine the level of chemicals your hair can endure. If your hair snaps when stretched out, it's too fragile for any straightening. I don't recommend you do this type of chemical process at home—leave it to the experts at your favorite salon.

As I've mentioned, almost all curly hair is baby fine—so please don't abuse it! We've come a long way since the days of torturous straightening chemicals that burn our hair and scalp. I've developed a system called Softening, which is very similar to straightening. The difference is the percentage of sodium hydroxide and the manipulation of the hair. A 4 to 8 percent concentration of sodium hydroxide (versus the 11 to 13 percent found in traditional relaxing and straightening) is blended with my

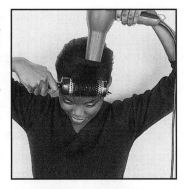

Deep Treatment to soften the hair without stripping the life out of it. I customize the percentage and ratio of the ingredients for each client.

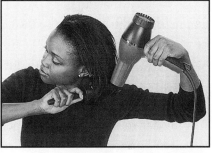

I prefer Softening to the more intense alternative, Relaxing, for two reasons. First, it forces the stylist to be attentive to the client— he or she should never leave your side during the process, because frequent manipulation is required to reshape the curls as the chemicals take effect. Psychologically, I also think the term *softening* reinforces kinder and gentler treatment.

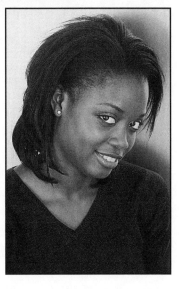

Stiff-straightened hair is

typically the result of Relaxing. In this approach, an 11 to 13 percent sodium hydroxide solution is applied directly onto the curls, which are then pressed to literally squeeze the life out of them. The whole process makes me sad, and yet the one who winds up the saddest is the customer. So please, stop!

One alternative to the harsh percentages of sodium hydroxide are new relaxers made of calcium hydroxide. Although the addition of calcium hydroxide makes the procedure milder, it doesn't soften the cuticle enough to smooth it out after the treatment, so the hair remains swollen and vulnerable to dryness and breakage. Calcium hydroxide is acidic and makes hair even more brittle. I've found it's better to use a very low percentage (from 4 to 8 percent) of sodium hydroxide than expose your hair to further damage.

Whether you choose a harsh straightening process or a gentle softening service, remember that any chemical treatment dehydrates the hair. So don't forget to use a deep conditioning treatment every two weeks.

Dear Ouidad,

I'm forty-three years old, and my curly hair has always been a problem for me. I gave Roseanne Rosannadanna a run for her money! One day I decided to have my hair straightened. I hounded my stylist during the process to make sure to keep the chemicals on long enough, because my hair has always resisted attempts to straighten it. After three hours, my hair was flat as a board, and I couldn't stop grinning. I walked back to my office swinging my hair with glee. Everyone at work was staring at me. I thought they were shocked by the tremendous change, but in reality they were stunned because my hair was falling out in clumps! I didn't realize this until my husband told me at home that night. I frantically tried to call my stylist, but the salon was closed. I had to wait until morning to return to the salon for emergency conditioning treatments. I wound up losing 50 percent of my hair. I had to wear a wig while it grew back! I'm lucky I met you a year later!

Katherine L., San Francisco

Avoid tress stress by following these tips on how to prepare for the straightening process:

1. Prepare your hair with weekly deep conditioning treatments at home for a month to maximize tress condition.
2. Make sure the salon you choose uses a straightening formula with 11 percent or lower sodium hydroxide.
3. Ask your technician to mix in some conditioner with the chemicals to protect your hair. (It won't change the process at all.) Your stylist will customize the ratio of sodium hydroxide to activator and conditioner.
4. Don't shampoo the day of the straightening or the day before—just dampen your hair and apply deep conditioner before going to sleep. This ensures extra protection for your hair from the chemicals.

THE SALON SMOOTHING PROCESS

1. Your stylist will apply the customized blend of sodium hydroxide, activator, and conditioner with a fine-textured application brush. (It looks like a paintbrush.)

2. The stylist will apply the mixture to the tightest curls first, to allow maximum exposure and time for the smoothing process.

3. The stylist will make sure your entire mane is saturated with the chemical formula, then allow several minutes for the cuticle to swell and become pliable.

4. Using a wide-toothed comb, the stylist will manipulate your hair into the desired wave pattern, to soften the S shape of your curls. This process will be repeated every few minutes. Make sure your stylist doesn't leave your side during this time.

5. Depending on the level of straightening, the chemicals will stay on your hair for seven to fifteen minutes. During this time, you'll actually see the hair relax and drop into softer curls. When your tresses feel bouncy to the touch and fall into the desired curl shape, you're home free.

6. Your hair will be rinsed with a neutralizing shampoo to close the cuticle.

7. Request a deep conditioning treatment to further seal the cuticle. You'll need to sit under a hair-dryer with low heat for about twenty minutes to help the conditioner penetrate. If this isn't possible, do an at-home treatment.

8. Get your hair cut. Now that the shape of your curls is completely different, you'll need a new style to accommodate it.

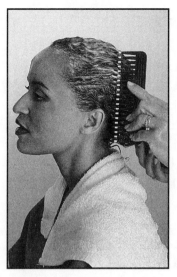

THE SMOOTHING PROCESS

AFTER THE SALON

1. Maintain smoothed-out locks with a low-pH shampoo. Many companies list pH on the label—look for 7 or lower.
2. Avoid massive heat styling. Use a cooler setting on your blow-dryer, and don't overdo it with the hot rollers, curling iron, and so on.
3. Stay away from alcohol-based styling products and all mousses. These will dry out hair and make it really fragile.
4. Be gentle! Think of your hair as an autumn leaf that can easily crumble.
5. Straighten, then color or perm hair. Wait ten to fourteen days between any two chemical services.
6. Don't skimp on deep conditioning every two weeks, especially in the summertime.
7. Minimize exposure to the sun, as with any chemical process. (Wear a hat, or coat your tresses in deep conditioner when you spend time outside.)
8. Your newly softened locks will stay smooth for three to five months. Repeat the process approximately three times a year for tight curls and once a year to relax softer curls.

TO COLOR OR NOT TO COLOR: YES! YES! YES!

Hair color is no longer a secret shared between a woman and her hairdresser. Today women are banging down their colorists' doors begging for highlights, touch-ups, and bold new looks. Even the media have taken notice of this movement, broadcasting funny commercials about using hair color on buses and in courtrooms and singing its praises in elevators. The last time I was in Paris, I even noticed women shopping at the outdoor fruit market while their hair color processed. I love it! The next time I color my hair, I'm going to do the whole procedure on a New York sidewalk by the salon. My clients always run down to the corner deli while they're in the midst of processing, so why can't I flaunt it? Okay, maybe that's getting a little carried away, but at least it's clear people are having fun with their hair color.

The bottom line is, I'm a huge fan of hair color—and so are 80 percent of American women of all ages. Hair color rates as equally important as the cut itself, and with the right tones, it can enhance your features tremendously. Most women are still using hair color to cover gray, but the number of women experimenting with completely new shades and innovative techniques is quickly growing. Men also turn to hair color to conceal their grays, and some even add highlights to create an ultranatural, multihued effect.

Although hair color is a chemical process, just like straightening, the procedure has several benefits. One of the main advantages is its ability to add incredible shine to tresses by sealing and thus smoothing the cuticle. Because curly hair is multidimensional, it doesn't shine the way flat, straight locks do, and so it thrives on the added glisten factor. Another bonus is texture: although curly hair often seems voluminous, individual strands can be quite fine and droopy. Hair colorants fill the cuticle and offer a boost to limp locks.

Most important, curly hair retains hair color better than any other type of hair. Why? We're back to the basic structure of curls: the corkscrew shape keeps the outer layer open, so the hair shaft is often empty. Gentle, semipermanent colorants, which normally coat the exterior of each strand, can instead deposit pigments into the hair shaft itself. This means the color will behave more like permanent hair color, looking more vibrant and lasting longer, but without the harsh side effects. Permanent color normally must break down the cuticle in order to penetrate the hair shaft. On curly hair, the lifted cuticle allows the color to fill the hair shaft without risking breakage and dullness.

All forms of hair color are dehydrating to curly hair—no matter how gentle the formula is, so Feed! Feed! Feed! Three days before coloring your hair, apply deep conditioning treatments to give the strands substance and to allow the colorants to absorb evenly. Ten days after coloring, repeat the deep treatment to keep the color molecules bonded and to prevent fading.

If you're ready to have some fun with hair color, let me guide you through the color services that are best for curly hair and answer a few common questions.

CHOOSING A COLOR

It's best to stay within two shades of your natural color. Women who try to dramatically lighten dark hair without the use of a peroxide lifter will wind up with orange tresses. (A lifter is a form of peroxide that removes the color from your hair before the newly desired shade is applied.) You can color your hair any shade you wish, but remember: the lower the strength of the activator (the ingredient that makes the chemical process of coloring occur), the longer the color will take to fill up the hair shaft with pigment. Just make sure you don't overprocess your delicate curls. Always work with semipermanent colors and gentle formulas—they will add shine, enhance your natural color, and coat your mane, taming it of frizz.

THE BEST COLORS FOR YOUR CURLS

In addition to matching your hair color to your skin tone, it's important to find a shade that works well with your curl pattern. The right color can add shine, dimension, drama, and lots of fun to your look. Loose curls are flexible and look great with a wide variety of colors. Take your primary cues from your complexion, and then the sky's the limit—fireball red to platinum white! Medium curls are fabulous with multihued highlights. This gives your curls terrific play and dimension. If you have a dark base color, don't get carried away with light blondes and caramels—these pale shades will wind up looking like frizz. On the other hand, light hair allows for more playful looks, so try reds, caramels, blondes—anything will look good. With kinky curls, work with tone-on-tone shades that add depth—you don't want to stray too far from your base color. A radical color change demands harsh chemicals and will damage these tender locks. If you're set on a major change, keep your hair short to minimize exposure to these intense chemicals.

HIGHLIGHTS

Although all hair types can be highlighted, curly hair reacts best to colorant-based, not bleach-based, highlights. The open position of a curly hair cuticle leaves the hair shaft exposed and vulnerable to damage from a harsh chemical such as bleach. Small streaks of different colors are less aggressive on the mane and look more natural. The range of shades scattered throughout the tresses adds lots of dimension to the hair. And fortunately, this is a single-step process. In terms of colors, brunettes should choose reddish and warm golden tones. Lighter-colored highlights will brighten up the wave pattern for a fabulous effect. Of course, for chemically processed hair, use a gentle activator, and Feed! Feed! Feed! I strongly discourage double-process highlights, which require lightening the hair before bleaching the specific streaks. Curly hair is too delicate, and intense doses of chemicals will only weaken and dehydrate the tresses, leaving them damaged and vulnerable.

COLOR GLOSSES

One color process I recommend and use is a vegetable gloss. It offers tremendous shine and comes in a wide range of colors, made by the top professional brands such as Redken, Sebastian, and Paul Mitchell. A vegetable gloss works well on absorbent curly hair and lasts for up to six weeks. To accommodate everyone's busy lifestyle, I suggest choosing a gloss close to your original shade so the hair color washes out naturally and won't create a tacky demarcation line as your roots grow in.

BLEACHING

I don't recommend bleaching unless you are 100 percent aware of the damage, time, and money involved. Curly hair is so delicate that stripping it of its natural color is like taking a gun and killing it. Unless you're an actress or singer who demands this harsh process, stay away! If you do bleach your hair, its only chance of survival is for you to condition, condition, condition! Even then, I can't promise you won't have breakage.

HENNA

Henna is a natural color derived from plant roots—and dirt! Henna and curly hair don't make a good combination because the cuticle fills with dirt and builds up until the hair shaft feels like cement. Overuse of henna will clog the hair shaft and make the hair feel hard and unpliable. Henna also spoils the natural curl pattern and volume. I won't mention names, but I once tried to remove henna from a Parisian actress's hair when she tired of the red color. I spent an entire day and even resorted to paint thinner and could not rid her hair of henna— the strands were as hard as a rock! Finally, we had to cut her hair very short to eliminate the problem. The moral of the story? Everything natural is not necessarily good!

DO-IT-YOURSELF

Forget about it! Coifs always look better when colored by the hands of a professional. Most processes are too complicated to try at home and still produce decent results. It's also very difficult to touch up your own roots. A trained expert will help you choose flattering colors that complement your skin tones.

Very often, do-it-yourself hair color will not mirror the shade shown on the box. At-home formulas are typically not as effective, durable, or vibrant as salon hair color. I realize many of you don't have the time or money to visit a salon regularly, so if you take your hair into your own hands, be careful! Home hair color always comes in two parts—the developer (the milky creamy liquid) and the tube of color. Follow the instructions carefully, and then try my trick: Dump out one-third of the developer, and replace it with water to make the formula gentle enough for tender curly hair. But please leave the heavy-duty jobs for the professionals. Don't say I didn't warn you!

Here are a few home hair-color kits I recommend:

* Clairol Natural Instincts (all hair)
* Clairol Hydrience (all hair)
* L'Oréal Féria (all hair)
* L'Oréal Casting ColorSpa
  (for covering a little gray and adding shine)
* L'Oréal Open Color Gel
* Garnier Nutrisse with Fruit Oil Concentrate

COVERING GRAY

I have many clients with beautiful gray hair. Personally, I love natural silver-gray hair, but you have to have enough of it to create that striking look. Generally, the darker the hair, the more graceful the graying process. So most of the time I talk clients out of coloring their gray. But with hair that's light in color, from light brown and red to blonde, tresses look dirty until they're completely gray and benefit from transitional coloring. Another good candidate for coloring is fine, thin hair that ages the face. In both cases, I suggest lowlighting, a process using foils to weave that "pepper" shade into salty locks. This is a semipermanent hair color and simply requires longer processing time. When necessary, I use heat to encourage the color to deposit into the hair shaft. A colorist may also choose to comb in the dark shades to create the look you desire. Traditional highlighting is another great look for gray manes, especially when the colorist blends many shades into your original color to provide the most natural effect.

The simplest way to mask gray hair is to darken it with semipermanent color. But gray tresses often resist this process. If that's the case, ask your colorist to add a little activator to the formula to help the color deposit properly without damaging the hair. To change gray hair to a lighter color, you'll need to add a "lifter" to the color. Remember, gray curly hair is especially porous, which means it acts like a sponge, changing color very easily. Be careful when exposing your hair to powerful chemicals and harsh products. For example, chlorine has a tendency to turn gray hair green. Smoke-filled rooms and overuse of curling irons and hot blow-dryers lend a nice yellow haze to your grays. Purple and blue shampoos produce that "sweet old lady" lilac tinge to your locks. To avoid these carnival colors, keep your hair clean and well conditioned.

Tip: Regardless of who cuts your hair, make sure to schedule appointments every three months unless you're in the process of growing out hair color or going through a straightening process.

Curve Balls!
Special Issues with Curly Hair

CURLY HAIR AND KIDS

Whether you adore your own curls or still view them as a challenge, I beg you to sing the praises of your children's curls! Your child hears your disparaging remarks and sees your face filled with frustration—great fuel for low self-esteem. Work with your children to have fun with curls, and view them as special, not troublesome.

As a mother, I want to share my experience with other parents. When my sister and I were little, we would visit relatives with my mom. Before we'd leave home, she would say, "Now let me see if I can do something with that hair." It sounded so hopeless and horrible, as if it were a tremendous problem we had to face. My sister and I now joke about that saying, but back then it crushed us! Our self-esteem really took a beating and always needed time to rebuild. I see the same issues reappearing in the salon today with successful adults. They complain about how they need to control their hair and how their mothers had such a hard time with their hair that it was always tied back.

Whenever a mom walks into the salon with her daughter from age four to the teenage years, my guard goes up immediately. I listen carefully to the words the mother uses to describe her daughter's hair and their frustrations. Here are some memorable quotes:

* "Look at her hair." (delivered with such a look)
* "Have you ever seen anything like it?"
  (said with eyes rolling to the ceiling)
* "Is there anything that can be done?"
  (voiced with exasperation)
* "Poor thing, she got stuck with it."
* "We don't know where it came from."
* "Do you think it will change, as she grows up?
  She can't go on with the rest of her life like this!"

Moms and dads, your curly-haired daughters have not been cursed—they've been gifted. As you come to understand curly hair, you'll find how easy it is to handle. Please be careful of the messages you send your children—some of us have been scarred for life by thoughtless remarks. In the salon, when I sense a mother is going in a negative direction, I stop her and ask if she'd be kind enough to give her daughter and me some private time to discuss her hair. I also speak separately to the mother about the hurtful messages she may be sending out. Inevitably, the mother's face is filled with guilt, and she immediately turns apologetic to her daughter. My entire staff is on Mom Alert—but we know not all moms are like that. But all moms (and dads!) do slip once in a while.

THE RIGHT WAY TO HANDLE CURLY KIDS
A child's curls do not need to look like Shirley Temple; nor do they require hours of work. Keep in mind that your child's

waves are new to the world and are not environmentally damaged the way an adult's are. Just as you wouldn't put a full face of makeup on a toddler, you wouldn't load up his or her hair with styling products. Keep it simple. The only time you'll need serious help from styling products is if your child has thick, fine, and tight curls, in which case a good lotion will provide control while some pomade will keep the frizziness at bay. Keep in mind that a child's hair texture will change three times before age twenty-one. Every seven years the body chemistry changes, and you'll witness a new curl pattern—so don't be surprised when your old "tricks" no longer work. Just adapt to the change, and don't fight nature!

I have firsthand experience with young curls—those of my daughter, Sondriel. From the day she was born until her current age of ten, I've used tender loving care on her gentle waves. I wash her hair every two to three days with ultra-mild, detangling shampoo. I condition her hair each time I wash it, leaving 25 percent of the conditioner on the ends after I rinse. On the days we don't shampoo, I still spray leave-in conditioner and a tiny bit of gel to tame her hair. With this routine, her hair is ready to go, whether we clip, tie, braid, or put it up.

MYTH: *Curly hair is inherited.*
TRUTH: Yes and no. Take my family: while my sister and I have always had curly dark hair, my two brothers have curly blond hair. My father had wavy blond hair, and my mom had very curly red hair. If there are lots of curls in your family, you're more likely to have curly hair or curly-haired children, but it's unpredictable—just like the curls themselves. The bottom line is, curly hair is a way of life, not a temporary con-

dition! Once you've made peace with those wavy locks, your life will be much simpler.

MATURE HAIR

Mature hair develops over the years as your color pigments weaken and fade. The hair becomes dull and has a light, tinny cast to it. It is extremely porous and acts like a sponge (which is terrific for hair color . . .). Mature hair appears in two textures, wiry and lacking pigment, or fine and limp. Although neither category sounds appealing, the two different textures complement and support each other.

GRAY HAIR VERSUS MATURE HAIR

Not all gray hair is mature hair. Just recently I attended my aunt's eightieth birthday party, where I was bound to run into many relatives I hadn't seen in years. It had been sixteen years

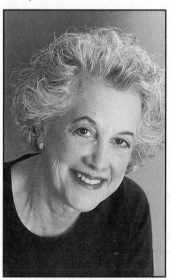

since I'd seen one of my cousins, now in her early forties. In that time, she lost her child to a sudden death. This shock manifested itself in her hair—it had turned completely white. When I first saw her from behind, I thought she was her mother until she turned to face me. This type of hair is not considered mature—it is new hair that grew in without any pigment as a result of emotional stress.

My cousin's hair is actually quite gorgeous—a bright, shiny platinum shade that many women would pay to have done in a salon.

ADAPTING TO GRAY HAIR: CUT AND COLOR

It's important to adjust to your new hair color and texture. Your previous haircut, styling techniques, and colors may not translate to your gray hair, so why fight it? I love a well-cut healthy head of silver curls—it looks sophisticated and regal. Of course, it's not for everyone—it takes a certain attitude to pull off a crown of platinum. In fact, you need to be at least 60 percent gray for this look. Anything less than that will make you look tired and age you unnecessarily. If this is the case, go ahead and color it—there are many terrific professional and home hair colors that work with gray.

Gray hair looks best in extremes, so consider a chic short cut or a stunning cascade of long curls. Whatever style works for you, remember to limit your exposure to high heat from the blow-dryer, which can singe the tresses and give them a mousy, yellowish cast. If this happens, wash your hair with Clairol's Shimmering Light Shampoo, which eliminates the yellow tinge from the blow-dryer, smoke, or sun.

DAMAGE FROM CHEMICAL TREATMENTS/ GROWING OUT STRAIGHTENED HAIR

Surprise! Chemical-free hair is healthier and less expensive to maintain. The real challenge is achieving healthy hair when, after countless visits for coloring and perming, you can't remember your original hair color or your true wave pattern. Patience is a key virtue in this process.

GROWING OUT CHEMICALLY STRAIGHTENED HAIR

As you know, I believe the best route is the path of least resistance, so I recommend starting over. No, don't shave your head! Wait until you have approximately three inches of growth—this will take about three months from your last chemical service. There's no point in trying to work with half a head of damaged, fragile hair and half virgin regrowth. It's impossible to run a comb through this dual-textured hair, and it will only invite more breakage.

If you don't want to cut your hair short to eliminate the damaged sections, it's possible to make the transition more gradual. Cut layers into the overprocessed hair, and slice it in a way to create movement as it grows out. For this process, I recommend a trim every two months instead of the usual three months.

If you find your straightened ends are too stiff and the new growth is kinky-curly, use the blow-dryer to straighten the newer hair to blend the whole mane together. See your stylist for trims every six weeks to get rid of those damaged ends little by little. To avoid further damage—Feed! Feed! Feed! Monthly deep conditioning treatments are essential to protecting your tender new hair as it grows. If your hair is especially dry and damaged, step up the treatments to every two weeks.

Another method for handling "the stiffs" (the stick-straight ends) is to curl your entire mane with rollers, braid it, or—if you're desperate—use a curling iron. Normally, I discourage the use of curling irons because they singe the hair, but in growing-out situations, I look the other way. If you resort to the curling iron, make sure to use it on the ends only—do not touch the new growth with this damaging appliance!

One other tip is to apply daily conditioner on your ends prior to shampooing. While washing your hair, place the shampoo on the roots only. As you lather and scrub, avoid the ends. As you rinse, the conditioner will protect the ends from further dehydration.

GROWING OUT HAIR COLOR

If your hair has been bleached or permanently colored, chopping it off is your easiest path, although this route is not realistic for many of us. To manage a bicolored look, consider these options. If your hair is bleached, you can add lowlights (darker streaks of color instead of the light ones used in highlights). Choose a shade close to your natural shade, and weave this tone into your hair gradually. Yes, this will mean several trips to the salon—it is definitely a job for your colorist. An instant overhaul rarely looks right. Another helpful step is to apply a deep conditioning treatment onto bleached hair to nourish it and allow it to hold the color better. Follow it with a colored rinse close to your original hair color.

For dark hair that's been lightened with a permanent color, make the transition with a semipermanent formula that is closest to your natural shade every eight to ten weeks until your hair grows out. (If the contrast between your new and original shade is extreme, use the semipermanent color every six weeks.) For hair that's dyed black, you can return gradually to your original color by weaving lighter shades into it with foils. This process will lift the black out and allow you to deposit the lighter semipermanent color onto these sections. Be sure to weave lots of light sections into your hairline to soften your look as you return to your natural color. And of course, Feed! Feed! Feed! The trip back to healthy hair is arduous and requires lots of deep conditioning to rebuild the strength of each strand. Don't forget, your hair is your crowning glory!

HAIR AND SCALP CONDITIONS

As if it weren't challenging enough to care for our curls, several special conditions may require extra treatment. The fragile condition of curly hair leaves it more vulnerable to certain scalp and strand issues and equally vulnerable to harsh remedies. It's important to be gentle with your curls and to consult with a physician when addressing solutions.

ALOPECIA

Alopecia is thinning hair, female pattern baldness, and sudden hair loss. In my twenty-six years of experience, I've seen countless women endure all of these conditions. My first advice is to see a doctor immediately, because alopecia is the result of severe stress, trauma, infection, heavy medication, or serious disease and requires a medical solution. A poor hair care routine, including abusive heat styling and chemical processing, can also cause massive hair loss. Once the problem is diagnosed, most women will experience regrowth in approximately one month. If the hair falls out leaving round bare patches, the condition is called alopecia areata. The hair will grow back in about six months.

DANDRUFF AND DRY SCALP

Both itchy scalp and white flakes are extremely common skin conditions caused by the increased production of skin cells. Many if not all of us battle this flare-up as a result of stress and seasonal changes such as cold, dry winters. Don't try to solve this problem by oiling your scalp. All the moisturizers, ointments, and conditioning treatments won't ease this itch. Instead, try using an over-the-counter dandruff shampoo that contains zinc pyrithione, tar, or salicylic acid. Of course, if none of these formulas work, consult a dermatologist. Ordinarily, I don't recommend harsh dandruff shampoos for tender curly heads, but there is nothing worse than ugly white flakes in your hair. Focus the shampoo on the scalp, and don't create a thick lather. Follow the cleansing with a deep conditioning treatment on the body and ends of your hair without touching the scalp.

ECZEMA

This itchy scalp rash will not cause hair loss but can encourage horrific scratching that will cause breakage. Cortisone creams work wonders, but it's best to speak with a dermatologist for a complete diagnosis and treatment.

PREGNANCY

When you're pregnant, your entire body is on overdrive. After giving birth, your estrogen level drops abruptly, and your body goes into shock. Having been there twice myself, I can report firsthand that my curl pattern went haywire postpartum, and my hair is now thinner than it was before both pregnancies. It wasn't until I cut and restyled it that I could work with my new wave pattern. Some of my clients have lost up to 30 percent of their original hair, which made it quite hard to handle. I tell them to be patient—as their eyes throw daggers at me—and then I have the nerve to continue the conversation! I believe it takes the same amount of time to con-

ceive and carry your baby as it does for your hair to return to
its previous self. In the meantime, be kind to your hair and
yourself. Use a protein-based moisturizing shampoo and conditioner, and apply a deep treatment frequently to revitalize
your hair. And as I always say, Feed! Feed! Feed!

MYTH: *Curly hair becomes straighter with age.*
TRUTH: As time goes on, our bodies experience many
changes. Curly hair doesn't actually become straighter, but
the curl pattern changes. With age we lose more hair, which
means our curls adjust into a less voluminous configuration.
Many women experience a similar effect after hormonal or
metabolic changes such as pregnancy, menopause, and dietary
shifts. The key is to adapt to the change instead of pretending
everything is still the same—good advice for all situations!

NUTRITION

We all know: we are what we eat! I hope this book is also teach-
ing you that you must feed your hair the way you feed your
body. The very best thing you can do for yourself is to eat
healthy foods rich in vitamins, minerals, and proteins, such as
leafy green vegetables, fresh fruits, grains, soybean products,
meats, poultry, tofu, fish, nonfat yogurt, and nonfat cottage
cheese. And don't forget to drink lots of water. On the other
hand, crash diets and marathon fasts can result in iron defi-
ciencies that can lead to hair loss. Anorexia and bulimia also
affect the condition of your hair: these illnesses make hair
sparse and finer in texture, and they change its color. Once
you resume eating well, your hair will return to its normal condition.

Dear Ouidad

Dear Ouidad,

I feel as though I have three different hairstyles—the sides and front are wavy, the layers underneath are tight, kinky curls, and the top layer from the crown down the back is straight, damaged, and strawlike. How can I care for my hair and attend to each section without damaging the others? Is there a haircut that's best for my situation?

Dear Reader,

Your situation is not uncommon. The first thing you need to do is find a knowledgeable hairdresser who can cut and blend all three hair textures. The straight section underneath should be cut and sliced shorter in modified layers, while the front and sides can be sliced for more movement around the face. A bit of carving in the tight crown area will help your curls "puzzle" into each other and lie flatter. If this still leaves you with a bulky look, I would recommend a softening treatment to tone it down and provide more "bend."

You'll need to break your styling into three sections as well. Apply gel on the straight lower layers, and give it a little curl during the drying process. Use a small amount of gel on the front and sides, and then let them be—no touching, no primping. On the tough crown area, apply gel section by section so each curl is defined. While directing the diffuser on them, pull down on these curls to stretch and loosen them. Finish the look with a light application of pomade.

———————————————————★———————————————————

Dear Ouidad,

I left your salon looking fabulous, with the best haircut of my life, but a few days later I couldn't reproduce your masterful styling techniques. What am I doing wrong?

Dear Reader,

Don't be frustrated! I've had over twenty-five years of experience working with curly hair—it's my job to make your curls look fabulous. Do you take the time to give your curls the attention I do? Probably not. Naturally, the solution is practice. You're not going to look like you walked out of a salon the first time you try to style your own hair. You should have seen some of the awful creations I made when I was first perfecting my techniques. It may take several tries, but once you've mastered it, the process is easy and will take only five to ten minutes. The key to salonlike styling for curly hair is to section the hair correctly. Make sure every strand is evenly coated with a light styling lotion, then create four to six sections of hair. One client suggests dividing the hair, applying lotion thoroughly, then flipping your head over and separating each section into perfect curls.

When clients complain that they can't re-create what was done at the salon, I have them come in and style their own hair while I watch. Nine times out of ten the problem is rushed and insufficient sectioning and gelling. So please be patient—you can do it!

———————————————————✦———————————————————

Dear Ouidad,

   What is your opinion of hair extensions on curly hair?

Dear Reader,

   Hair extensions are fun and blend in well with curls. I often use them on women with hair thinning at the crown by weaving in sections that are the same color and texture as their own hair. I love adding wild and trendy extensions in crazy colors on performers for concerts or creating new looks for actors playing roles with a specific look. One of my stylists, Ana, wins the prize. She loves extensions and appears at the salon with a different look every week!

———————————————————✦———————————————————

Dear Ouidad,

   Can you recommend an elegant style for my sister, who has dreadlocks to her waist? She's going to be in my wedding party, and she needs a more conservative look for that day.

Dear Reader,

   First, it's important to acknowledge the time and work involved in creating a head of dreadlocks. You may find the look messy and unkempt, but your sister is no doubt proud of her efforts. As for styling, you have a few options. On short hair, gel and twist each individual piece—work them all together or allow each piece to fan out slightly. On longer hair, gel each piece separately and gather all the sections at the nape for an elegant effect and a strong statement. Another option is to pull back the hair into interlocking twists for an elaborate style. The ends can remain sticking out, or you can create a loose ponytail and pin the "tails" up to create a design on the back of your head.

Dear Ouidad,

My hair is acting differently since we moved. We used to have hard water, and now we have soft, treated water. Could this be the problem, and if so, what can I do?

Dear Reader,

When you impose a new environment (and water) on your hair, it may act differently. The first step is to apply a deep conditioning treatment to fill your locks with moisture—providing the hair with nourishment while it adjusts to the new conditions.

Both chlorinated pool water and city pipes have a tendency to cause mineral and copper deposits on the hair, while salt water can cause dryness, severe tangling, and breakage. Well water can leave iron salt on the hair and turn it red! To battle these problems, always rinse and condition your hair immediately after swimming in a pool or the ocean. To protect the hair from well water and city pipe water, leave a little extra conditioner on your hair after shampooing. I also recommend using a shampoo with the ingredient disodium EDTA, an agent that helps attract and lift the minerals away from the hair shaft. Follow this cleanser with a generous dose of conditioner—it will act as a neutralizer.

Dear Ouidad,

I told my hairdresser I wanted some softness around my face instead of this head of massive, thick, curly hair. Her solution was to cut off the hair around my face and give me bangs. I hate them. What should I do?

Dear Reader,

My sympathies to you. I am not a fan of bangs either. With curls, bangs never stay in place, and they look incongruous when blown out straight. The good news is that because your bangs are curly, they can blend into the rest of your hair easily during the growing-out process.

The only time bangs look right with curls is when the entire mane is sliced into a curly shag. Just keep in mind that the shortest piece of hair around your face should stretch from the top of your forehead to the chin. This allows enough length to accommodate shrinkage, provide movement around your face, and complement your facial structure.

Dear Ouidad,

Why do I lose more hair than my straight-haired friends?

Dear Reader,

You and your friends lose the same amount of hair, but it falls out differently. One strand may fall out in your hair, but it remains trapped in your curls until you comb or wash it. Your fallen hairs collect and make their appearance all at once—usually in your shower drain! When straight hair falls out, it immediately drops to the ground, so you don't see the same accumulation as you do with curly hair.

Dear Ouidad,

I feel as if I must choose between working out and having beautiful hair. Every time I go to the gym, I know I'll leave with frizzy, awful hair. Am I destined to be either out of shape or out of style?

Dear Reader,

Go with the flow, and don't fight nature. I assume from your woes that you're attempting to preserve straightened hair. The humidity your hair experiences from perspiration will turn your smooth locks to frizz in no time. Instead, start the day by drying your hair in natural curls with a diffuser and a healthy dose of defrizzing gel. Not only will your curls look great, they'll be hydrated and impervious to the frizz-producing moisture from your workout.

Dear Ouidad,

No matter how much gel I use and how much time I spend, I can't control my hair.

Dear Reader,

Controlling your hair is a matter of quality and technique. First, find a breathable styling gel that is free of curl-stifling silicone. This will allow your waves to look lively and healthy. Second, try my styling method—apply a small amount of gel to the hair to reduce the tiny flyaway hairs, then divide your mane into small sections. Apply more gel to each section in order to create smooth, defined curls.

Dear Ouidad,
  Every time I diffuse-dry my hair, it frizzes!

Dear Reader,
  Don't use the diffuser on soaking wet hair. Apply your gel, and let it sit for at least fifteen minutes before hitting it with the blow-dryer on medium heat. Also, make sure you are directing the heat from underneath your locks, not on top. This will prevent the fine baby hairs on the surface from becoming flyaways and frizz.

Conclusion

Now that you've read my book, I hope that you have a better understanding of how to work with your curls. Wear them proud—they are your crowning glory! As I'm saying this, I have an image of all my clients smiling . . . and rolling their eyes! But no matter how corny I get, they know I've proven to them that curls are an asset. Now let me prove it to you. Try all the tips I've given you—don't be intimidated. They sound time-consuming and difficult, but they're not. Be patient—you may feel "all thumbs" the first few times, but with practice you'll zip through my styling technique in just five to ten minutes. I have a client who can divide her hair into six sections, apply gel on each, flip her head over, use her fingers to separate the curls, and then finish off with a light hairspray in *five* minutes!

I can help you with the external factors—the cut, the styling techniques, the appropriate products—but it's your job to change your attitude. How you *feel* about your hair matters more than anything. We all know if you don't look good, you really won't feel good no matter what anyone says. Probably every woman has had at least one very bad day with her hair or a horrible experience with it. You can wear the top designer dress with all the jewels in the world, but if you don't have your hair together, you will never look together or finished. I know I've had more than my share of those moments—and that's how my passion came about.

I'd been fighting this curly hair battle all my life until one day I realized that I really don't have a battle to fight. I have a life to live. So here I am: a woman at the top, living life to its fullest just like my hair—proud, shining, spunky, friendly, and fun. So take my experience, my clients' stories, and my foolproof tips and tricks, and make peace with your curls!

Index

ABOUT THE AUTHOR

OUIDAD is an author, stylist, trainer, educator, wife, and mother. She is the founder of the Ouidad Salon in New York City—the only salon in the country that caters to curly hair. She is the creator of her own hair care line, distributed worldwide, and continues to research, formulate, and produce new and current products. In addition to extensive media appearances and speaking engagements, she is regularly quoted in national women's magazines about curly hair. Curly-haired celebrities often seek out Ouidad for consultations and styling sessions.

Ouidad is cofounder of a direct response company. Her website, www.ouidad.com, is a resource for women with questions and concerns about their curly hair. She also trains other salon affiliates nationwide in curly hair techniques.

She shares her home in southern Connecticut with her husband, Peter, their son, P.J., and daughter, Sondriel.